Start Well!

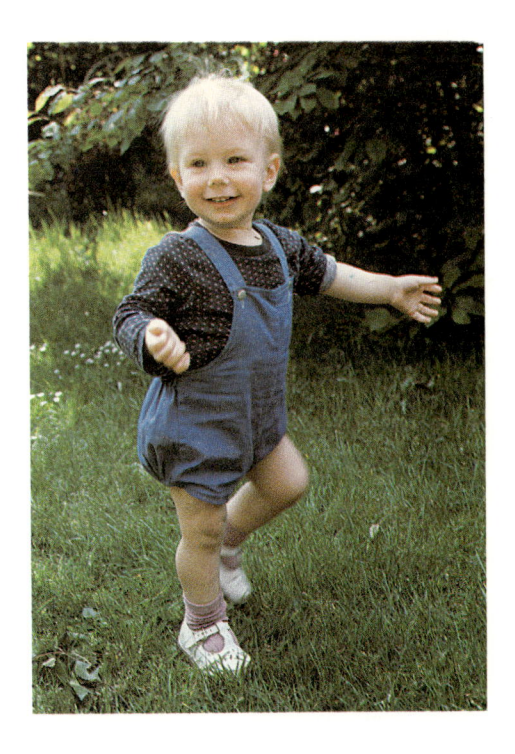

To everyone who inspired and
helped us to write this book,
we offer our thanks.

Michael and Inke Schwab

Contents

PART 1
A good beginning

	Pages
Conception	8–9
From embryo to fetus	10–11
Diet in pregnancy	12–13
Guidelines for a balanced diet	14–23
Taboos and temptations	24–25
The nutrients in pregnancy	26–27
The micro-nutrients in pregnancy	28–31
Energy, calories and weight gain	32–33
Overweight and underweight	34–35
Diet and pregnancy problems	36–37
To breast or bottle-feed?	38–39
Feelings about breastfeeding	40–41
Preparations for feeding	42–43
The birth	44–45

PART 2
Feeding the newborn

Early feeding	48–49
At the breast	50–51
More about breastfeeding	52–53
The diet and breastfeeding	54–57
Early bottle-feeding	58–61
The mother's well-being	62–63
Your baby's digestion	64–65
Early feeding problems	66–67
Weight gain	68–69

PART 3
The weaning process

Growth and development	72–73
A flexible weaning program	74–77
A new balance	78–79
Illness and diet	80–81
Dietary deficiencies	82–83
Supplements, rhythms and routines	84–85

PART 4
Appendix

Mother's nutrition notes	86–87
Baby's nutrition notes	88–89
Glossary	90–91
Cookbooks	91
References	92–94
Index	95–96
Useful addresses	96

Start Well!

A Guide to Healthy Eating for You and Your Baby

Michael and Inke Schwab

Managing Editor Susan Pinkus
Production Manager David Alexander
Photographic Coordinator Siân Phillips
Administration Aline Davis, Sonia White
Editorial Assistants John MacRae-Brown,
　　　　　　　　　　　Dusica Radovic
Glossary John Rivers
Design Behram Kapadia

MICHAEL and INKE SCHWAB met in Paris in 1973. Inke, having obtained degrees in German and sociology at the Sorbonne University, was working as a journalist. Michael, a nutritionist, was researching into French eating habits. They married soon after and now live in Berkeley, California with their two sons Daniel and Luc.

Michael Schwab has an M.Sc. in nutritional science from London University, and has worked as a researcher in the field of psychosomatic eating disorders; as a local health education counselor in England; as a company nutritionist in the baby food industry; and as a consultant for international food agencies in Africa and the Caribbean.

Inke Schwab has spent most of the last ten years with her family. During her first pregnancy, she worked as a freelance translator and tended a vegetable garden. After her second pregnancy, she began teaching pre- and post-natal yoga. The first birth was in hospital; the second, at home. She breastfed both children for two years.

The Publishers gratefully acknowledge the cooperation of all those who have so kindly given assistance with the illustrations featured in this book.

Photography by Anthea Sieveking

Artwork by Design Practitioners Limited

Text copyright © 1984 Michael and Inke Schwab
Compilation and design by Pagoda Books, London

All rights reserved. No part of this publication may be reproduced, stored in a retrieval system or transmitted in any form or by any means, electronic, mechanical, photocopying, recording or otherwise, without the prior permission of the publishers.

NOTE
While the authors' aim has been to provide a good basic guide to nutrition, from pre-conception to weaning, the advice contained in **START WELL!** is not intended as a substitute for consultation with your own doctor.

ISBN: 0-86683-846-5
Library of Congress Catalog Card Number: 84-50005

Origination by East Anglian Engraving Co. Ltd.
Typeset by Design Practitioners Limited, Sevenoaks, Kent
Printed in Great Britain by Blantyre Printing and Binding Co. Ltd.

Introduction

The information presented here by Michael and Inke Schwab is set, as it should be, in the rich fabric of parenthood and in the totality of early child development. They do not prescribe a nutritional pathway that promises salvation to those who follow it, nor do they threaten those who stray. Instead they offer up-to-date facts to parents who wish to be well-informed, as well as sensible practical guidance for those who are bewildered by the variety of opinions currently offered on nutritional matters. This is an exciting and interesting exposition of the vital part that nutrition has to play in the emotional and physical life of the mother and her child.

I hope that their enjoyable message will reach and influence many prospective and actual parents. It can also be read with profit by professionals who advise on nutrition and who all too often fail to take a broad view.

THOMAS E. OPPÉ
Professor of Pediatrics
St Mary's Hospital Medical School, London

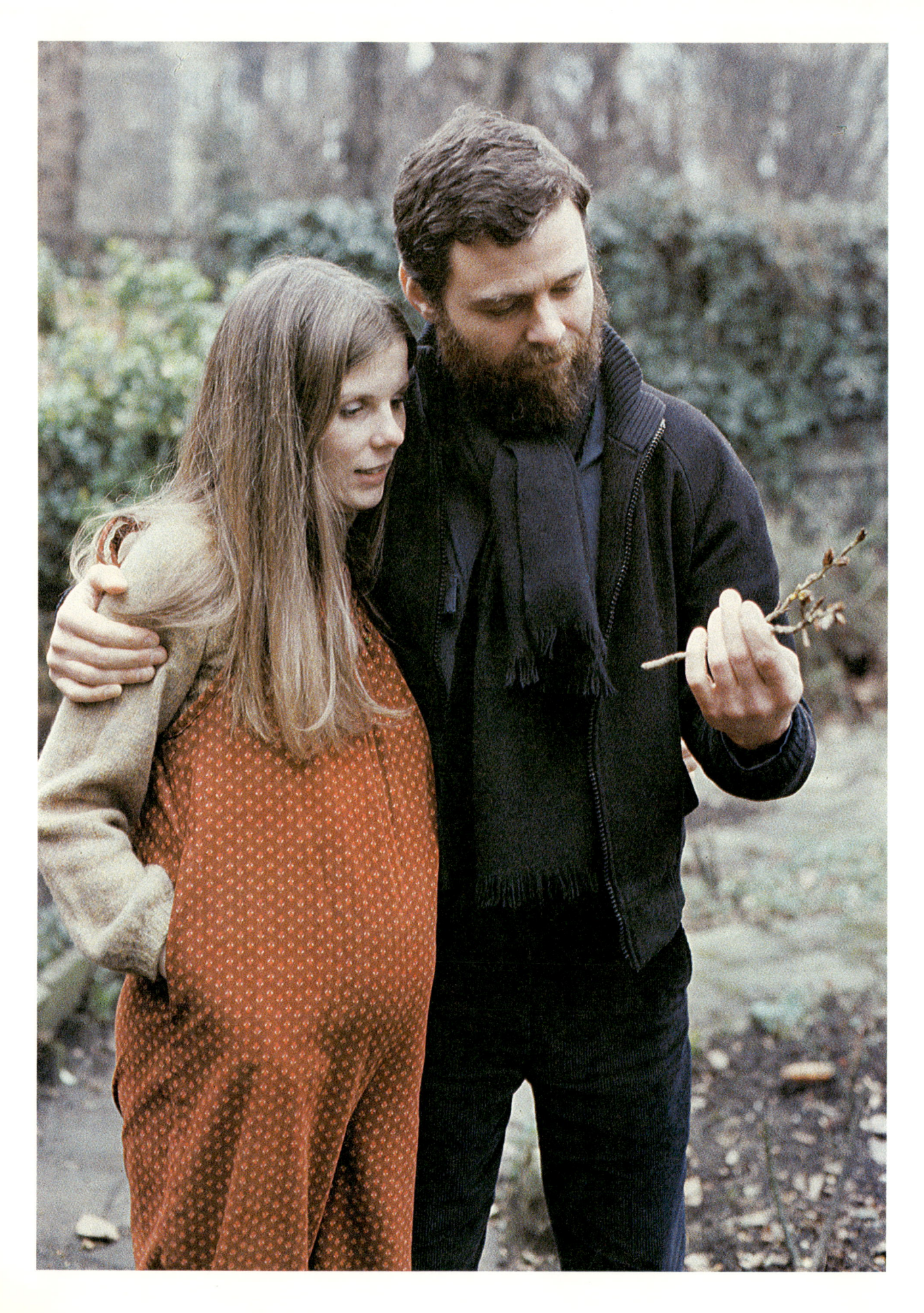

PART 1

A good beginning

The flow of life from generation to generation is maintained by two things: food and love. We reproduce, we nourish ourselves and each other, we excrete our wastes to the earth and the sea, and finally we follow them. For millions of years, humans have been making love and conceiving children. At least two hundred thousand generations of mothers have nourished their offspring in the womb, at the breast, and eventually from the family cooking pot. Yet each generation sets about the task in its own way.

What we eat has a profound effect on our health: and if you are pregnant, your diet influences not only your own well-being but also the health of your developing baby, just as the quality of the soil affects the plants that grow in it. To some extent, your diet may even affect the kind of birth you have and, after the delivery, may influence the quality of your milk.

Later still, when you embark on weaning, it is what *you* eat that largely decides what *your child* learns to eat. This is the natural process. Nor is this strong link between a mother's diet and her children's health limited to the years in which she starts a family. For what you were eating *prior* to conception – even the way *you* were fed in your mother's womb – may affect your baby's growth and development. Recent research has shown that the father's diet, too, may play a vital part.

Conception

We begin at the beginning with a man and a woman making love, their bodies flushed with *oxytocin*, one of the so-called 'hormones of love'.[1] *Hormones* are the chemical messengers that our bodies use in the biochemical regulation of life as it flows through us, a regulation so precise and so astonishingly adaptive to the changing world that we can sometimes only wonder at it.

At the climax of love-making, four hundred million male seeds rocket through the vaginal canal towards the woman's womb: male seeds looking for the female egg. The journey is a perilous one. After an hour, barely a thousand have survived to reach the woman's Fallopian tubes which lead from the womb to the ovaries. If she is fertile, there may be in one of these tubes, slowly descending according to the woman's monthly cycle, an egg, one female cell, a sphere two hundred times the size of a sperm cell. The minute seeds vibrate around the comparatively massive egg until one is permitted to penetrate. Leaving its tail outside, the fertilizing sperm is swallowed up.

The female egg or *ovum* is largely composed of food, a rich gelatinous mass of nutrients that will nourish the fertilized egg once it begins to grow. It also contains a nucleus, its 'biological computer', programmed over thousands of generations with details of how a human body is built. Like the nucleus of the fertilizing sperm cell, it carries information on many family characteristics, both physical and mental, encoded in its genes. When the two nuclei of the male and female cells unite, conception takes place.

Food and health

For every living creature, from conception to death, food plays a vital role in health. Every cell of your body needs to be nourished, to provide energy for daily life and to help repair damaged tissue. When cells naturally wear out, as they constantly do – blood cells, for example, last only ninety days – it is food that supplies the raw materials for their replacement. Muscle and bone cells, nerve and brain cells, the cells of inner organs, sperm and egg cells, hormones and *enzymes* (which catalyze chemical reactions within the body): all need a constant supply of nutrients to carry on their work.

The *type* of food you eat, and how you eat it, also affects the efficiency with which you breathe and think, work and play; the ease with which you are able to withstand stress, and your ability to resist disease. If you generally eat the kinds and amounts of food you *need* (which may not always be exactly what you *want*), your chances of good health will be high. If, on the other hand, you consistently eat too much or too little – either of food or of any vital component in food – your diet will be unbalanced, increasing the chances that you will feel run down, become depressed and be subject to infections. Poor nutrition can also affect your love-making and can even prevent conception.

Science, following in the footsteps of common sense, has now established beyond any doubt that a woman's ability to conceive and nourish a child is profoundly affected by what she eats, not only during pregnancy but also in the years before.

Diet before conception

There are many factors that influence whether or not conception will occur: a woman's age, her genetic inheritance, her general health, the nature of any previous pregnancies, her desire for a child, and her diet. All are important.

At worst, malnutrition – which usually means insufficient intake of food, although it can also refer to an unbalanced diet – will actually prevent conception. At a very low threshold of food intake, however, conception is not prevented. Nor is it necessarily prevented by any but the most unbalanced of diets. Throughout the Third World, malnourished women conceive with awesome regularity.

But for those babies who are conceived despite a poor diet, the risks of abnormal growth and development are definitely higher than for the babies of well-fed women. Studies undertaken during and after the blockade of Holland during World War II show that women who conceive despite malnutrition bear an abnormally high rate of stillborn, premature and low birth-weight babies, and infants with permanent physical and mental handicaps.[2,3] In general, malnutrition at the time of conception and soon after is associated with physical abnormalities called *congenital defects*, while malnutrition in later pregnancy – when the baby's physical development is virtually complete but growth is still rapid – tends to result in low birth weight.[4,5,6,7]

Nor are the effects of malnutrition before conception necessarily limited to the first generation: animal experiments suggest that it may take several generations to reverse any damage done. Sometimes called the 'granny effect', this phenomenon has been demonstrated in mice and rats, where a third generation may have a learning impediment as a result of the poor nutrition of the first generation.[8] Retardation becomes progressively more marked with each generation that lacks adequate food.[9]

When malnutrition is less severe – not starvation as in war-time Holland but, rather, an unbalanced intake of foods – the effects appear to be similar. Most of this information comes from work on laboratory animals. Rats given a diet complete in all nutrients except Vitamins A or E, or the minerals *zinc* or *magnesium*, become sterile until the appropriate supplements – or foods containing those missing nutrients – are added to their food. If only low levels of the missing nutrients are added, the rats conceive but have a high rate of congenital defect in their offspring. If a balanced diet is fully established with adequate amounts of *all* the nutrients, healthy development is restored.[10]

It is certainly important to eat not only *enough* food, but also a *balance* of different foods that provide enough of all the nutrients. Exactly what constitutes a balanced diet is a ticklish question that takes up a large part of this book. But as a general principle, we can say that if you are planning a family and have been eating a lot of white bread and pasta, processed meats and sugary foods like cookies and colas, now is certainly the time for a change!

As a woman, you are not alone in this, for a man's diet may also play a part in the events of conception. His sperm production, like the rest of his health, is affected by what he eats, and severe deficiency of either Vitamin E[11] or zinc[12] may reduce the number of viable cells so that conception is less likely to occur. Male sterility can result from a number of environmental poisons, too, like cadmium and lead, against which a good diet offers some degree of protection. Severe lead poisoning, for example, as a result of continuous exposure to lead over a long period, can cause abnormal sperm and either sterility or – if a baby *is* conceived – congenital defects.[13] Foods rich in zinc and iron (like wheat germ, liver, nuts and seeds) and in Vitamin C (like oranges and other citrus fruits) are in some measure protective against lead poisoning.[14,15]

The diet of either parent before conception may, according to some schools of thought, also affect the sex of the child, which appears to be decided at the moment of conception. The evidence is scanty but the idea is an old one. Dr. Leopold Schenk, in his treatise *The Determination of Sex* (1898), propounded the view that sweet foods eaten by the parents may lead to the conception of a girl, while saltier foods are more likely to result in a boy. This is somewhat in line with the traditional Japanese view that a diet of *yang* (salty) foods give boys, while a diet of *yin* (sweeter) foods may give girls. A more up-to-date version of the theory is proposed by Professor Stolkowski in Paris, who suggests that parents who eat a diet rich in *sodium* and *potassium* (meat, beans, artichokes and apricots, for instance) are more likely to conceive boys, while those who stick to foods rich in *calcium* and *magnesium* (dairy products, eggs and green vegetables) are more likely to have girls.[17] His evidence is far from conclusive, but the theory is not unreasonable.

Stress and drugs

The modern world is full of potential stresses that we adapt to the best we can. Air pollution, noise, economic difficulties, and high unemployment, fear of nuclear war, and a rapidly rising divorce rate are among the pressures of life in the 1980s. To cope with these stresses, we have turned, as a society, to drugs of one kind or another. Addiction to alcohol, tobacco, hard and soft drugs, to pharmaceutical medications, to coffee, tea, and even to sugar (which is also addictive) has become commonplace. All these substances alter the body's chemistry and our state of mind, helping us to cope for a while but, in the long run, making us less able to manage. For prolonged use undermines good health. Regular heavy smoking and drinking are well-established causes of abnormal growth in pregnancy, and so is heavy caffeine intake. Sugar is also related to a number of conditions that can disrupt pregnancy, such as diabetes.

In the West, between five and ten percent of all babies are born with some physical or mental handicap, often mild but sometimes severe. Although retarded growth in the womb can sometimes be reversed in a good environment after birth, many of these babies have lifelong disabilities. *Now* is the time to lay good foundations for your family, preferably *before* you become pregnant. If you have been unkind to your system, *now* is the time to change.

The process of kicking the habit is made much easier if you can find other, less self-destructive ways of coping with life. Millions are taking up swimming, yoga, jogging, or stretching because such exercise helps us feel well and remain relatively unrattled by the stresses of everyday life. And the effects run deep. Twenty minutes a day of hatha yoga postures, for example, will slow the heart rate, deepen breathing, reduce blood pressure, and increase flexibility[18] – all effects that can help you in pregnancy and childbirth.

The regular use of any kind of drugs, because they alter the way the body works, also tends to alter nutritional requirements. This is also true of the contraceptive pill which, with regular use over several years, appears to deplete the body of (or increase requirements for) a number of micronutrients, including Vitamin B_6 and E, and the mineral *copper*.[19,20,21,22] So, in pregnancy, eat plenty of whole grains, nuts and seeds, which are rich in these nutrients. Your doctor may also recommend a low-level multivitamin and mineral preparation if you have been using this form of contraception.

From embryo to fetus

The fertilized egg, the *blastocyst*, floats down the Fallopian tube to the womb, dividing and sub-dividing as it goes, drawing nourishment from its own gelatinous store of nutrients and from fluids secreted by the Fallopian tube and the walls of the uterus. These are the first foods of your child-to-be. But the store will soon be spent. The blastocyst cannot absorb all it needs from the surrounding fluids, so it must anchor itself to a more abundant source of food. On the seventh day, it lands on the rich inner surface of the uterine wall and slowly implants itself, sinking into the tissue.

Within hours, the fertilized egg begins to tap the uterine blood vessels for food, and the more it can draw off, the better its chances of survival. If the egg is implanted – as is normal – in the upper rear portion of the womb, where the blood supply is especially abundant, the embryo will grow well. But occasionally, an egg will implant in a part of the uterus where the blood supply is poor. This limits its chances of optimal growth.

Once implanted in the uterine wall, the growing blastocyst becomes an embryo, and now takes on the rudiments of human form. What remains of the original food store in the egg becomes the yolk sac, a private 'larder' that takes about four weeks to empty, at which point it becomes the embryonic digestive tract. By the time this happens, there is a strong flow of nutrients directly from the mother's blood to the embryo.

A month after its conception, your child-to-be has a head, a spine, the buds of arms and legs, and a heart, as well as blood vessels delivering food to all parts of its body. At ten weeks, all the essential inner organs, including the digestive system, are formed and most of them beginning to function. These early months are subject to a delicate and specific biological timetable; and any major interference may result in abnormality.

The placenta

Quite early in pregnancy, the outer cells of the blastocyst combine with cells from the uterine wall to form the *placenta*, an all-important spongy, oval, blood-rich organ that serves as a sort of 'guardian' for the developing baby. Firmly anchored to the uterine wall and connected to the baby by the three strands of the umbilical cord, the placenta both nourishes the unborn child and receives its waste products throughout the pregnancy. After its nine months' work, it will be born with the baby, before being separated and abandoned as the *after-birth*.

A fascinating organ, the placenta receives the blood of both mother and baby. The mother's blood flows into the maternal side of the placenta, where selected nutrients are screened out and transferred to the baby's blood which carries them along the umbilical vein. This process is known as *placental transfer*. The nutrients all come from the mother's blood and are derived either from her diet or from her body stores. Waste products are transported back from the baby to the placenta along the two umbilical arteries.[1]

Though there is an exchange, in the placenta, between the blood of the mother and that of the baby, each maintains a measure of independence. They are always separated by a barrier within the

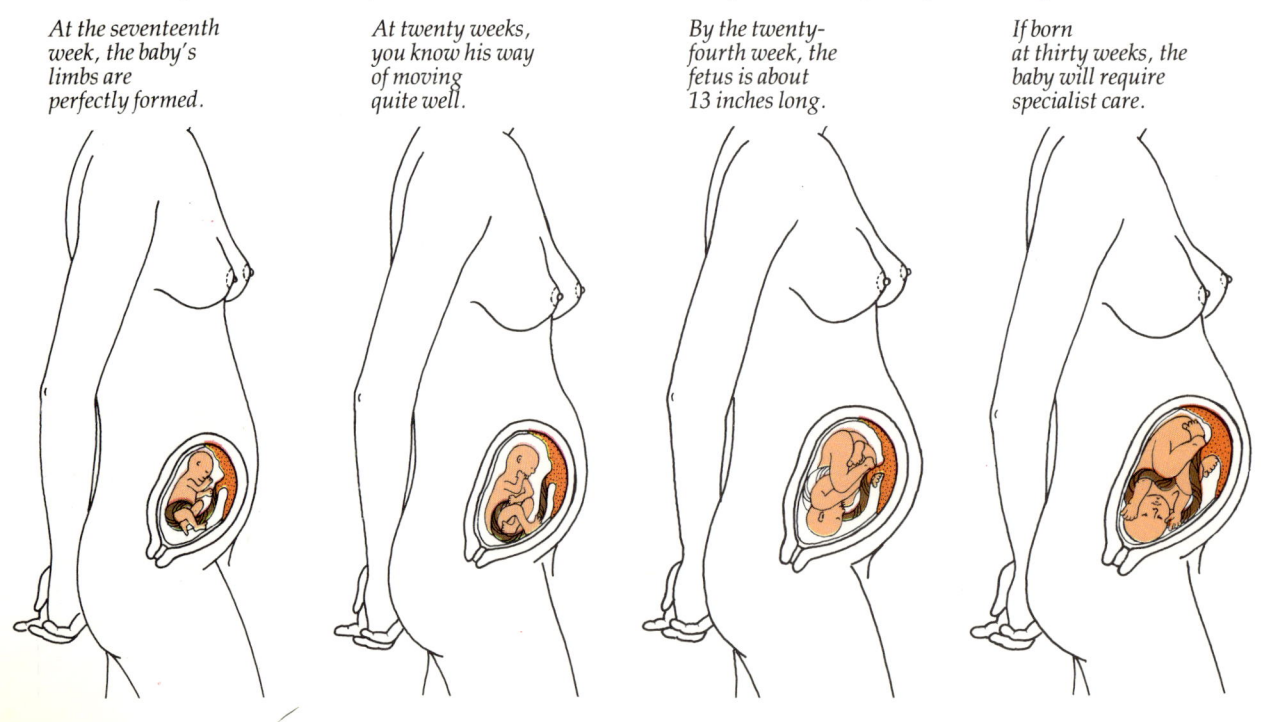

At the seventeenth week, the baby's limbs are perfectly formed.

At twenty weeks, you know his way of moving quite well.

By the twenty-fourth week, the fetus is about 13 inches long.

If born at thirty weeks, the baby will require specialist care.

From embryo to fetus

placenta. It is this barrier that 'selects' the nutrients needed from the mother's blood whilst preventing, to some extent, the transfer of potentially harmful substances. As it is the baby's blood which flows through the umbilical cord to the placenta and back again, a part of the baby's blood system is always outside his or her body. This would appear to explain the view of the British psychiatrist, Francis Mott, that the fetus in fact consists of both his own body *and* the placenta, with these two parts being separated when the cord is cut soon after birth.[2] Certain societies in Australia, the Pacific Islands, Africa, and the Americas even treat the placenta as the newborn's 'other soul' or 'little brother', burying it reverently after the birth, with much gratitude for services rendered![3]

Maternal adaptation

As soon as you become pregnant, your body rapidly adapts to the presence of the blastocyst. Stimulated by hormones, your heart – which sends blood to your lungs for oxygen before pumping it down the arteries to the rest of your body – starts to work more efficiently. It even enlarges in order to increase its output, since additional blood is required to carry nutrients to your breasts, to fat stores in your thighs and of course to the uterus. In fact, a pregnant woman's blood volume virtually doubles by the birth.

To provide additional nutrients for both you and the baby, your digestion also adapts to the pregnancy. The rhythmic, peristaltic contractions of the intestine slow down so that they empty less rapidly, thus enabling greater absorption of nutrients from food into your blood. The kidneys – which regulate the blood composition, removing excess water and nutrients into the urine – also adapt by retaining certain important nutrients that are now needed.

Yet another adaptation seems to have evolved specifically to modify the mother's intake of nutrients: an increased sensitivity of hunger and appetite. Animals adapt to pregnancy with increased hunger, which makes them eat more, *and* by seeking out particular foods, as part of a more sensitive appetite. Humans are no different. Though there are always some pregnant women who feel like eating less than usual – especially in the early months, and particularly if they were overweight at conception – most end up eating more. And most also find themselves quite choosy about which foods they want to eat.

Development and growth

From the formation of the baby's first hard bones at about three months, the embryo has become a *fetus*. His body looks thoroughly human, although a few external parts – his eyelids, toenails, and genitalia – are still not quite complete. (We have two sons and so perhaps quite naturally refer to the fetus as 'he'). Floating weightlessly within the waters of the protective amniotic sac, he flexes his newly forming muscles, gently bumping against the side of the womb. His diet now comes almost entirely from his mother's blood, but he also swallows surprisingly large quantities of the amniotic fluid surrounding him, and this also supplies him with certain essential nutrients.[4, 5]

Gradually, as he starts to distend your abdomen and your clothes no longer fit well, you will become more and more aware of him. You may feel like caressing him by stroking and rubbing your belly; you may dream about him, you may even feel like talking to him. Don't feel embarrassed: there is somebody living inside you and all the positive attention you can give him will be happily received.

Indeed, your *attitude* towards the baby is one of the most important factors influencing his development and growth. Mothers who feel positive towards their pregnancy are much more likely to have an uncomplicated labor and a healthy baby than those who are negative. For the fetus responds to his mother, both physically and mentally.[6] At six months, he is sensitive to touch in most parts of his body and all his sensory systems are functional: he can see, hear, and feel you. Your ways of moving and talking are already being imprinted in his mind. Love him and feed him well now, and his pre-natal impressions will be good ones.

At thirty-two weeks, the fetus will weigh around 3½ pounds.

By the fortieth week, your baby is ready to be born.

Diet in pregnancy

A balanced diet in pregnancy increases your chances of delivering a healthy, fully-grown baby in an uncomplicated birth. It is not, as some enthusiastic writers would have you believe, a guarantee: there are far too many other factors at play for that. But a balanced diet throughout pregnancy will provide all the nutrients that your fetus needs for his development, and that you need in order to become fit for the birth, and for subsequent breastfeeding.

The first evidence of these effects of a good diet came through a number of studies undertaken in the 1930s and 1940s. Until that time, it had been widely assumed that provided the mother had enough to eat (in quantity), her fetus would simply take what he needed from her body. This notion of the fetus as a 'perfect parasite' was, however, challenged in 1934 by vitamin-research pioneer Professor Edward Mellanby, who believed that the *quality* of the mother's diet was at least as important as the *quantity*.[1] One of the first research reports to support this view came from the Canadian physicians Ebbs, Tisdall and Scott, who showed that the rate of premature births and of perinatal deaths among women who were assessed as having a poor diet could be reduced by giving food supplements. Among the supplemented women, the rate of successful breastfeeding was also improved.[2]

Other studies[3,4] added weight to Mellanby's hypothesis, including the long-term evidence of another Canadian group at the Montreal Diet Dispensary.[5,6] Here, it has been clearly shown that mothers who are given help in balancing their diet early on in pregnancy are less likely to deliver babies of low birth weight than poorly nourished mothers who do not receive dietary guidance. At the Montreal Dispensary, free oranges, milk, and eggs were made available to mothers considered to be at risk, thus providing a well-balanced, protein-vitamin-mineral booster to their normal diets. As we shall see, extra foods and food supplements need to be *balanced*: too much of one nutrient – protein, for example – can actually reduce the baby's birth weight and cause other complications, just as too little of certain nutrients may have harmful effects, too.

Those considered to be most at risk by the Montreal Dispensary were teenage mothers, especially those on unusual diets; women substantially underweight; mothers who have borne a child within the previous two years without eating well enough to replace lost nutrients; and those women with diabetes. Other stressful situations include those of the single mother and of the severely overweight woman. In all these circumstances, an unbalanced diet reduces the chances of a good pregnancy and a good birth.

Finding a balanced diet

But what is a balanced diet? We use the term so lightly, as if the answer could be supplied in a moment, yet every nutritionist seems to have his or her own idea of what is implied, as do many mothers, magazine health and beauty editors, infant food manufacturers, healthfood store owners, and restaurateurs. There is clearly no universal truth on the matter.

This may seem confusing. But it is in fact how it should be, given that we differ so widely in our individual requirements and tastes – not only in race and body-size, temperament and profession, but also from day to day and season to season. Individual needs for just one vitamin, for example, may vary ten-fold. So how are we to define what *your* balanced diet should be?

The vast majority of nutritionists take the statistical view. They use the official Recommended Daily Allowances (RDAs), which give the average amounts of each nutrient – the number of grams of protein and fat, for example, or the number of milligrams (one thousandth of a gram) of Vitamin C – that an 'average' man or woman theoretically needs each day to avoid becoming deficient.[7] A safety margin is added for those who may need more. But because the range of our *real* requirements is very wide and the RDAs are averages, this way of assessing a balanced diet can be misleading.

Another problem with RDAs is that they refer not to foods but to chemicals, the nutrients. In the hands of a skillful dietician, they can be converted into a weekly menu card, but for most people their value is limited. Even for the dietician, RDAs can be misleading, for the amounts of any nutrient in one kind of food may vary enormously. Two ounces of carrots, for example, may contain anything between 350 and 700 micrograms of Vitamin A (micrograms are one thousandth the weight of milligrams, which are themselves one thousandth of a gram) depending upon the soil and the season of their growth. As the RDA for Vitamin A is 750 micrograms, a two-ounce portion of carrots may provide anywhere from half to all the average daily requirements.

The RDAs have led to some very odd advice being handed out to pregnant women, even by otherwise responsible professionals. How many times have you heard that you need four glasses of milk a day when pregnant? And if you are under twenty years of age, and your body still growing, it is sometimes said to be six! Cows' milk was designed to provide for the rapidly growing calf: it contains far more protein and calcium than you are likely to need in pregnancy, and not enough of other nutrients, like Vitamins A and C. For many women, it also causes certain allergies.

It is not only milk that pregnant women are exhorted to consume in vast quantities: mountains of meat (especially liver), eggs, fish, dairy products, vegetables, and fruit – not to mention any number of vitamin and mineral supplements – are widely recommended. Fortunately, nature has provided a much better way for you to find a balanced diet – in the form of hunger and appetite, your own natural physiological signaling systems that tell you what and how much to eat.

Hunger and appetite

Hunger is a signal that food is required: a rumbling of the stomach muscles as they contract, a twinge as digestive juices begin to flow, perhaps a salivation of the mouth. The mechanisms involved in hunger have long been the subject of scientific debate. Blood levels of sugars, proteins, and hormones, temperature changes, and signals from the body's fat stores have all been proposed as messengers to the brain of a need for food.[8] Internal rhythms also play a part, especially those based on habitual mealtimes, and so do the wider rhythms of life – the seasons of the year and a woman's menstrual cycle, for instance.

The efficiency with which hunger can regulate food intake can be clearly seen in studies of breastfed babies. Fed whenever they appear to be hungry, these babies regulate their intake in direct proportion to their body weight,[9] and in direct relation to the composition of the mother's milk, which varies over a twenty-four hour cycle.[10] Heavier babies drink more than lighter ones (unless the lighter ones are 'catching-up' from a period of under-nutrition); and breastfed babies tend to drink more by day, when the fat content of the milk is relatively low, than by night.[11]

Young children, fed when they are hungry and not over-encouraged to eat when they are not, also show a clear understanding of when they need to eat.[12,13] The same is true for many adults and, because pregnancy is a particularly sensitive time, this includes a good many pregnant women, too. But there are also many who have lost touch with their true sense of hunger: they tend to eat out of phase with their needs, perhaps overeating, perhaps undereating.[14] At the extremes, these women are either obese or *anorexic* – that is, without appetite – and very thin.

Appetite – the drive to find and eat food or particular foods – is a more sophisticated mechanism than hunger. It contains an element of learning, based on past experience of what we have eaten and found acceptable. And a healthy appetite appears to be the process in which our physical needs for nutrients are converted into specific desires for foods.[15] The pregnant woman who craves pickles has become a traditional cartoon character, but there is every reason to believe that such a craving can actually be a signal that she needs some nutrient which her body has 'learned' is found in pickles. Both animals and young children can, as we shall see, select a balanced diet if a broad range of natural foods is available. In pregnancy, the same appears to be true for many women, for the appetite is likely to be working with heightened efficiency.

If you find yourself suddenly craving pickles or pineapple or a particular kind of cracker, try to make sure you get what you fancy. It may well be just what you need right now. Similarly, if you find yourself disgusted by tea, coffee, fried foods, or anything else for that matter, avoid it. It is probably bad for you right now. Many pregnant women rely on appetite as a guide to a balanced diet. If your appetite is working well, you could have no better guide.

Some women, however, cannot rely on their appetites. Their cravings are not occasional but obsessive and self-destructive. One woman finds she cannot stop eating cake, something she has perhaps never done before; another eats mountains of spaghetti with a fixed look in her eye; a third compulsively drinks pints of milk that she does not like but that she has been told is good for her; a fourth takes secret trips to the kitchen for a spoonful of laundry starch or to the garden for a handful of earth. When the object of the desire is not really food at all, this distortion of appetite is called *pica*. Obsessive, self-destructive appetite patterns can sometimes be traced to emotional or physical problems; sometimes the cause remains unknown. Whatever their origin, the result is to unbalance the diet, with excessive intake of one set of nutrients at the expense of another.

If you feel that your senses of hunger and appetite are intact and functioning well, we recommend that you trust your own feelings about what you eat. To be sure that you are not missing any particular nutrient, you may be able to arrange for blood or hair analysis. This can, to some extent, reveal abnormal nutrient levels in the body. A poor diet in the past or regular use of tobacco, alcohol, caffeine or other drugs (either medical or illegal) may have depleted your body of certain nutrients.

If, however, you feel you may have lost touch with your true feelings of hunger and appetite, now is the best time for you to find a way back to them. If you have been eating a lot of junk food, or if you cannot stop gorging (or dieting), be prepared to admit that you might have an eating disorder. You can start on the road to recovery right away by studying the *Guidelines for a Balanced Diet* that follow.

Guidelines for a balanced diet

There are many ways to get in touch with your own senses of hunger and appetite so that you can more intuitively select a balanced diet: fresh air, suitable exercise, yoga, meditation, and loving relationships all promote a sense of well-being and thereby help us to 'feel' more clearly. But for those who are not sure where to begin, or feel that they cannot yet trust their senses of what and how much to eat, some guidelines are required.

These guidelines are actually for everyone. They deal with the kinds of food that help you feel well and the proportions of each in the diet. What they do not tell you, however, is *how much* you should be eating. That depends on *you*. During pregnancy, you may need more than before, and after the birth you may need even more if you are breastfeeding: but only *your* body can say exactly how much you need at any one time. A summary of our six basic guidelines follows, together with a table showing the proportions of different foods we recommend that you include. Notice that the largest proportion should ideally be whole grains, with highly processed foods taking only a very small place in the diet. Plenty of fresh produce, and not too much of the protein-rich animal foods like meat and milk, are other important elements of a well balanced diet.

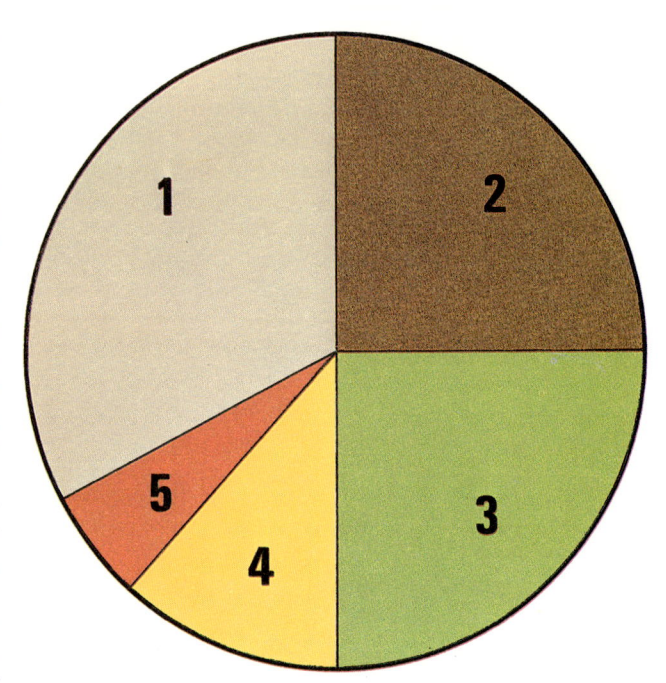

The key to a well-balanced diet is a matter of proportions.
1 whole grains; 2 animal foods, legumes and nuts; 3 fresh fruit and vegetables; 4 cooking oils and fatty spreads; 5 highly processed foods.

THE GUIDELINES

1. **EAT WHOLE GRAINS AS YOUR STAPLE FOOD**
   Wholemeal bread, wholewheat and rye crackers, corn-on-the-cob, brown rice
   Wholewheat or buckwheat pasta
   Oatmeal
   Wholegrain breakfast cereals and muesli (granola)

2. **ADD ANIMAL FOODS OR BEANS, SEEDS, AND NUTS**
   Lean muscle meat, e.g. poultry and beef (avoid fat)
   Meat organs, e.g. liver, kidney, heart
   Fish and shellfish
   Eggs, milk, and milk products, e.g. cheese and yogurt
   Legumes, e.g. soybeans, lentils, peas, beans
   Nuts and seeds, e.g. brazil nuts, almonds, sesame and sunflower seeds
   Nut and seed butter, e.g. peanut butter, sesame butter (tahina)

3. **INCLUDE PLENTY OF FRESH VEGETABLES AND FRUIT**
   Cooked root vegetables, e.g. onions, parsnips, potatoes, carrots
   Cooked leaves, e.g. spinach, kale, brussels sprouts, and cabbage
   Other vegetables, e.g. mushrooms, zucchini, and cauliflower
   Raw vegetables, e.g. tomatoes, cucumber, lettuce, and celery
   Raw fruit, e.g. apples, pears, cherries, plums
   Dried fruits, e.g. raisins, figs, dates, and apricots

4. **USE A VARIETY OF COOKING OILS AND FATTY SPREADS**
   For cooking: sunflower, safflower, corn, or olive oil; sunflower-rich margarine or butter for flavoring
   For salads: olive, sesame or corn oil
   For spreading: sunflower-rich margarine, butter, peanut butter, sesame butter, or soybean paste (miso)

5. **KEEP HIGHLY PROCESSED FOODS TO A MINIMUM**
   Cut down on sugar and foods containing sugar, e.g. cakes and cookies, ice cream, desserts, candy and soft drinks.
   Try to avoid very salty foods, e.g. potato chips, salted peanuts, salted cured meats and fish.
   Cut down on white bakery products.
   Try to avoid too many factory-made, pre-cooked foods that may contain harmful additives.

6. **TAKE YOUR TIME**
   Relax, try to enjoy preparing your meals and eating them in your own way.

GUIDELINE 1 Eat whole grains as your staple food

Wheat, oats, corn, barley, rice and rye are the main grains: the edible seeds of the grass family and the basic food of humankind for the last ten thousand years. In the Orient, rice is the staple grain; and in many poor countries, it makes up almost the entire diet. In the southern United States and in Central America, it has long been corn (maize) that holds body and soul together. In Tibet, it is barley. The Scotsman swears by his oats; the Scandinavians, by their rye. For all of them, the staple grain is an integral part of life.

The whole grain is complete: a seed ready to drop to the soil and reproduce itself. Like an egg, it contains everything required for the hatching out of the next generation. The 'yolk' of the grain is its yellow *germ*, the 'white' is its starchy *endosperm*, and the shell is its tough *bran* coating. The endosperm is the bulk of the grain, rich in carbohydrate and some protein. The germ and the bran are much smaller but have most of the vitamin, mineral, fat, and fiber content. All these nutrients are vital in our diet. When the grain is *refined*, so as to remove the germ and bran, a lot of these nutrients (and the taste that goes with them) are lost. Refined white bread, white pasta, and white rice – which are all made from the endosperm only – are tasty at times but a lot less nourishing.

In the developing nations of the Third World, grains still make up sixty percent of the diet, as they did for most of our great-great-grandparents. Among the wealthy, industrialized nations – and that includes most of Europe and North America, even if we do sometimes imagine ourselves to be poor – the place of grains in the diet has gradually been eroded by two other kinds of foods: those rich in oil or fat, and those containing sugar. In the West, we eat half the grains per head, twice the amount of sugar, and three times as much oil and fat as the average Third World inhabitant:[1] and of the grains we do eat, most are highly refined, not only into foods such as white flour and white rice but also – once fat and sugar are added to the mixing bowl – large quantities of cakes and cookies. The more of these refined carbohydrates you eat, and the less whole grains, the greater the chance that your diet will be unbalanced.[2]

The effects of an unbalanced diet are not always easy to identify, however. Early studies undertaken by pioneers like Robert McCarrison[3] and Weston Price[4] showed that societies changing to a highly refined diet develop a whole series of diseases within a generation or two: heart conditions, bowel problems, diabetes, and dental decay among them. McCarrison demonstrated that these diseases can be induced quite rapidly in animal experiments when the diet is radically changed, so it was clear that diet alone was a major contributory factor. Today we know that there are often other factors at play: for example, our genetic inheritance, overeating and smoking can all contribute to heart disease.[5]

You do not need to become one of those 'whole earth' people, endlessly baking bread over the kitchen range, nor do you need to follow an exclusively macrobiotic diet, eating mountains of brown rice and cutting out all refined foods. In fact, there is no reason for you to give up white bread, cakes, and ice cream *entirely* if you do not want to do so. There is even some evidence that a very *sudden* change from refined to whole grains may be harmful, since it can apparently take about three months for the digestive enzymes needed for wholewheat bread to become fully established in the intestine.[6] But if you have become used to eating a lot of refined foods, do try to cut down. A good part of your grains and cooking flour should be *unrefined*.

Wholewheat pastry (for pies, pizzas and quiches)
Makes a double 9-inch pie shell
1½ cups wholewheat flour
1½ cups white flour, unbleached
½ cup margarine/vegetable oil
½ cup butter (or margarine)
3–5 tablespoons water, cold
½ teaspoon salt

1. Having added salt, make a well in flour.
2. Cut the butter or margarine into small cubes.
3. Put the cubes and/or oil in the well.
4. Stir the salt into water and leave to dissolve.
5. With your fingertips, mix the flour and fat.
6. When crumbly, slowly add the salted water, kneading the mixture lightly into a dough that comes away easily from the fingers.
7. If dough is too sticky, add more flour.
8. Form into a ball, cover and store in a cool place for an hour before rolling out.

Brown rice (chewy, tasty and nutritious)
Serves 2
1 cup brown rice
2 cups water
¼ teaspoon salt

1. Place the rice in a saucepan, fill the pan with water, and stir the rice to liberate loose husks.
2. Empty water and rice into a sieve over the sink. Return washed rice to pan.
3. Add 2 cups of water and the salt, and boil.
4. Turn down the heat, cover the pan and simmer the rice until soft, for about 25 minutes.
5. Remove the pan from the heat and let it stand for 5 minutes to settle. Stir in a little butter to taste before serving.

Guidelines for a balanced diet

GUIDELINE 2 Add animal foods or beans, seeds, and nuts

Meat, fish, eggs and milk – the foods we get from the animal kingdom – play an essential role in most of our traditional dishes. They provide us with the raw materials for everything from sausages to soufflées. The trouble is that we in the West tend to eat too much of them, and many pay for it with poor health. Too much meat, butter, fatty cheeses, and eggs can, for example, not only make you fat but may also increase the risk of high blood pressure and heart disease.[7]

In the Orient and most of the Third World, animal foods are usually eaten in much smaller quantities. Legumes, seeds, and nuts, together with grains, provide the basis of the diet. Legumes are the family of peas and beans, the seeds of leguminous plants, which – when eaten with grains – are as nutritious as animal foods. For centuries, the Chinese have thrived on rice and soybeans, Moroccans on wheat and garbanzo beans, Mexicans on maize and red kidney beans, Russians on buckwheat and sunflower seeds, Malawians on corn and groundnuts, each group adding small amounts of fish or meat, vegetables, and cooking oil to their dishes. There are many combinations of grains and legumes, legumes and nuts, and grains and nuts that can form the basis of a well-balanced diet.

The *kind* of meat or fish, eggs or cheese that you eat also makes a difference to you health. The meat of animals raised in the wild or free ranging on a farm contains far fewer saturated fatty acids than meat from stall-fed cattle or from battery chickens.[8] Such meat is also free of the residues of antibiotics routinely fed to some farm animals.[9]

Fresh fish is another excellent source of nourishment, and by poaching, grilling, or steaming, you can minimize loss of nutrients during cooking. As for eggs and dairy products, enjoy them in all their abundant variety, but treat them as secondary foods in your diet, especially if you also eat meat or fish.

Baked trout
Serves 2
2 trout (cleaned, with heads)
2 teaspoons butter/margarine
1 teaspoon olive or sunflower oil
1 teaspoon parsley, finely chopped
salt and pepper
aluminum foil

1. Wash the trout, inside and out, under running cold water.
2. Dry the fish with a clean kitchen towel.
3. Season the inside of each fish.
4. Mix the parsley into two teaspoons of butter or margarine.
5. Stuff each fish with the parsley butter.
6. Melt the remaining butter/margarine and brush over each fish.
7. Sprinkle with salt and pepper.
8. Wrap each fish loosely in aluminum foil, twisting the edges to seal.
9. Bake for 30 minutes at 350° F in a pre-heated oven. When the gills come away easily from the fish, it is cooked. Remove the heads before serving the trout, if you wish.

Nut croquettes
Serves 2
1 cup peanuts, hazelnuts, almonds, filberts, sesame seeds, coarsely ground
1 cup soft breadcrumbs
1 teaspoon finely chopped mixed herbs (oregano, thyme, or parsley, for instance)
1 egg
1–3 tablespoons water
2 tablespoons flour
1 cup vegetable oil
½ teaspoon soy sauce

1. In a bowl, mix the nuts, breadcrumbs, herbs, soy sauce and egg. Moisten with water until slightly soggy.
2. Let the mixture stand until the water is absorbed. Roll into small croquettes.
3. Pre-heat the oil in a deep frying pan, but do not let it boil.
4. Coat each croquette in flour and fry lightly in the oil until golden brown.

You do not actually *need* to eat any animal food at all. Vegetarians manage very well omitting meat and fish from their diet, while vegans – who eat no animal foods whatsoever – can in fact be well-nourished on careful combinations of grains, legumes, nuts, and seeds. Milk and milk products like cheese, yogurt, and cream are excellent, nourishing, and convenient foods but they are not essential, even in pregnancy. The nutrients they contain can all be found in sufficient quantities in other foods.

If you enjoy meat, and have always done so, don't be persuaded that this is necessarily bad for you. Your family may have been eating meat for centuries and it may not be easy or even sensible for you to try and change too abruptly. *Some* change may, however, be a good idea. For animal production is ecologically expensive. An acre of farmland, for example, can be used to grow grains and legumes to feed forty people for a year, but the same area can provide enough animal food for only five people. In a world where the population is increasing by leaps and bounds and land is being farmed more and more intensively, we may need to get used to having less animal foods in our diet over future years, so that plant foods will have to take far more prominence.

Guidelines for a balanced diet

Follow the guidelines for a balanced diet: for lunch, maybe a fresh salad, wholewheat bread with egg and ham or cheese and fruit; tonight, perhaps, a dish of rice and legumes, like chickpeas or beans. Let your appetite be your guide.

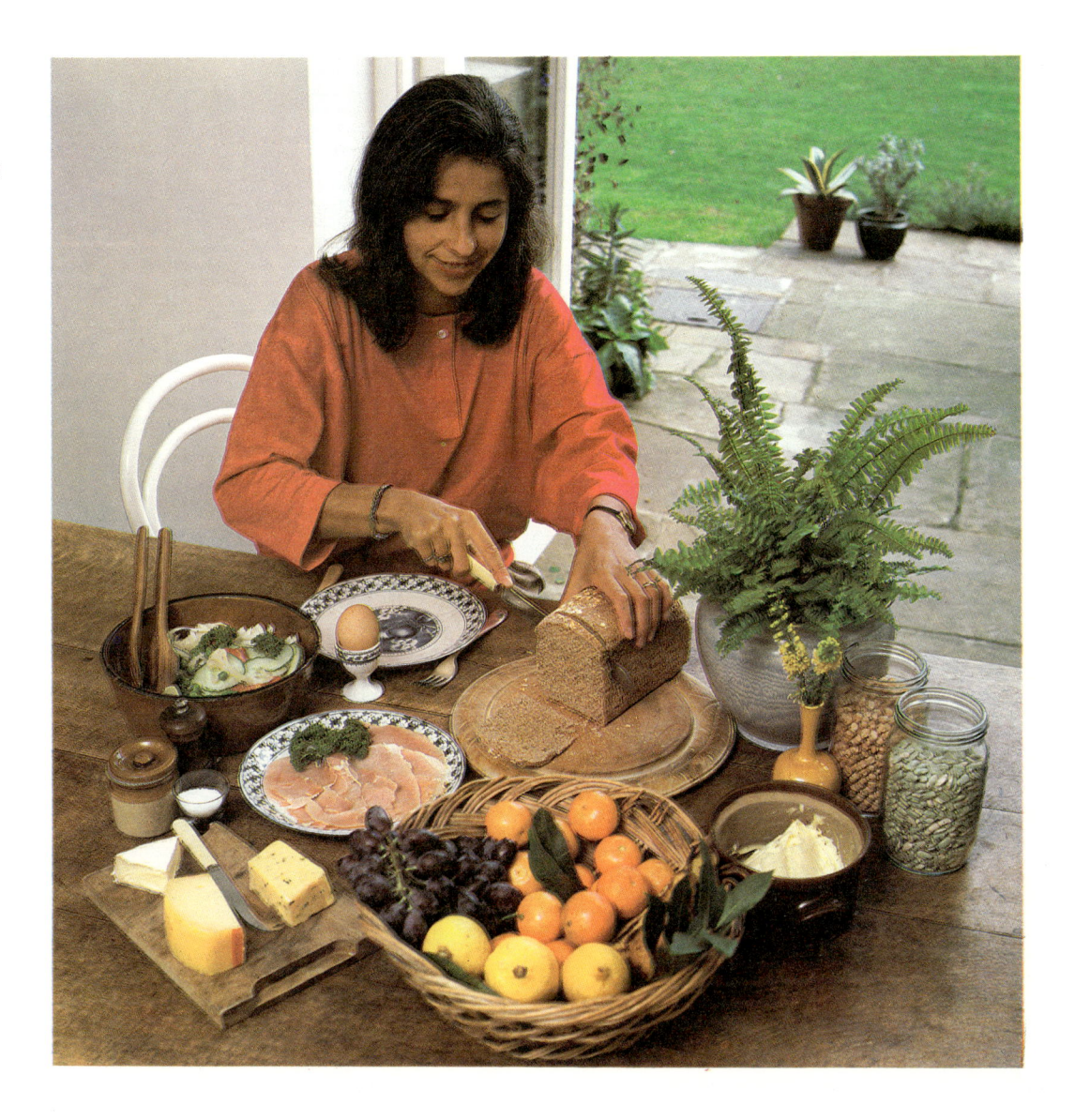

**Grains, legumes, nuts and seeds
in nutritious combinations.**
Wholewheat bread and peanut butter
Wholewheat toast and baked beans
Corn tortillas and chili beans
Peanuts and sunflower seeds
Rice and lentils
Wholewheat pita bread and chickpea
fritters
Bread with sesame butter (tahina),
and soybean paste (miso)

GUIDELINE 3 Include plenty of fresh fruits and vegetables

Vegetables and fruit should ideally make up about a quarter of your food intake: and because they contain up to ninety percent water, they can usually be added to the diet in generous quantities without any risk of overeating. They are a prime source of vitamins and minerals, and are sometimes called 'nature's own supplements'. Even potatoes – so often accused (quite wrongly) of making us fat – are highly nutritious if boiled or baked, rather than fried. They are in fact the major source of Vitamin C in many diets. Remember to peel them thinly in order to retain the maximum vitamin content.

Throughout your pregnancy, aim to eat some of your fruit or vegetables raw every day. We could try to explain the importance of this in terms of taste or texture or of nutritional value, but nothing so definite touches the essence of the matter. We could point to the sensible French tradition of starting the evening meal with crudités, a colorful platter of raw vegetables, including perhaps thinly sliced cucumber, chopped celery and finely grated carrot, beet slices and small crisp leaves of endives, all lightly dressed at the table. We can also remind ourselves that a salad containing nuts and seeds or cold cooked beans is, if eaten with a hunk of bread, a perfectly balanced meal in its own right. Yet there is something more in a meal like this. Perhaps it is that raw food is richer with *life* than anything cooked, and this is just what you need in pregnancy. We recommend that you eat a good mixed vegetable or fruit salad at least three times a week. There are so many exciting variations you can make to the basic salad.

Salad can also be a refreshing, colorful, nourishing snack, suitably light at a time when the rapidly growing uterus pushes against your stomach and intestines. As time goes by, you may well feel like eating several small meals or snacks a day instead of two or three larger ones. Make up a salad in the morning, and add dressing to a small portion whenever you feel hungry. A regular stock of mixed nuts, seeds, and dried fruits can also provide quick, very nourishing snacks. As an alternative, prepare a fresh fruit salad and add a juice prepared from lemon, water, and honey. Take a portion as a snack whenever you feel like it.

In general, if you grow your own or are able to buy in bulk, remember that freezing is a very good method of preserving the flavor and nutritional value of most vegetables and fruit. Some vegetables, however, are unsuitable for freezing because of their high water content, unless already part of a cooked dish. Among them are cabbage, green salad plants, cucumber, marrows, pumpkin, tomatoes and mushrooms. However, there will be no need to thaw most of those you can freeze before cooking. Most fruit is suitable for freezing, too, although strawberries may become very limp when thawed. So if you have a freezer, think ahead and you should be able to continue enjoying many vegetables and fruit even when they are out of season.

Cooked dishes of fruit or vegetables also freeze well: but many sauces and dressings have a tendency to separate when they are defrosted.

Cooked vegetables and fruit also add to a balanced diet. They give characteristic flavors and coloring to many of our favorite dishes, and form the basis of many more. What, after all, is a pizza without tomatoes, a roast without potatoes, carrots and onions, or a stew without peppers and garlic? True, some nutrients do tend to be lost in cooking, but others become more easily digested. So keep cooking your favorite dishes but also explore new ways of preparing vegetables so that any loss of nutrients is minimized. In general, the lower the heat and the shorter the cooking time, the less the loss will be. Some vitamins and minerals will inevitably be retained in the cooking water, and so these highly nutritious juices should also be used to form a stock whenever possible. The Japanese method of stir-frying vegetables – a quick fry and then a slightly longer steam in very little water – leaves vegetables cooked, yet still fairly crisp and rich in flavor. Steaming and baking are other particularly good low-loss cooking methods for vegetables.

Everyday salad
Serves 2
A colorful, infinitely variable combination of fresh, raw vegetables, for instance:
2 cups grated carrot, celeriac, radish
1 cup grated celery, cucumber, tomato
½ cup whole young corn kernels, peas
2 cups shredded lettuce, spinach, endive

For variety you can add one cup of any of the following:
orange or tangerine segments and grated apple
½ cup grapes, nuts, seeds
soaked raisins, prunes, and figs, as well as cubes of cheese

Wash and prepare your selected ingredients. Dress the salad, or a portion of it, before serving as an accompaniment to a main dish, or as a meal in its own right.

French dressing
6 tablespoons unprocessed olive, sunflower, or corn oil
2 tablespoons wine vinegar
pinch salt, pepper
½ teaspoon honey

Stir the seasoning into the vinegar. Slowly add the oil, stirring continuously.

Stir-fried vegetables
Serves 2
2 small onions, finely chopped
2 carrots, sliced thinly
1 cup cauliflower pieces
1 cup zucchini, sliced flat
3 tablespoons sunflower or olive oil
1 cup water or stock
1 cup grated cheese (optional)

1. Clean and prepare the vegetables, using a colorful mixture as above or with seasonal variations.
2. Heat the oil in a large, heavy pan or wok.
3. Add the onions and fry lightly until transparent.
4. Add the other vegetables and fry, stirring frequently with a wooden spoon.
5. Add the water or stock.
6. Season to taste.
7. Reduce the heat and simmer, uncovered, for about 10 minutes until semi-soft.
8. Serve topped with grated cheese, if liked.

Baked apples
Serves 2
2 large eating apples
2 teaspoons raisins or currants
2 teaspoons almonds or hazelnuts

1. Core the apples.
2. Chop up the nuts and mix with the raisins.
3. Stuff each apple with the nut-and-raisin mixture.
4. Oil a baking tray and place the apples on it.
5. Bake for 15–20 minutes at 375° F in a pre-heated oven.

GUIDELINE 4 Use a variety of cooking oils and fatty spreads

During the last three generations we, in the West, have doubled the amount of fat we eat each day. During the same period, the types of fat we eat have also changed with more and more coming from animals – not only in the form of meat but also as lard, cream, and butter. Only during recent years, as evidence has been produced to show that too much of these fats can contribute to heart disease, have we begun to swing towards using more plant oils and fatty plant foods instead.[10]

In general, the fatty plant foods – nuts, seeds, legumes, and the germ of grains – contain lighter fats than butter and lard. The oils of sunflower seeds, corn kernels, and sesame seeds have a high level of unsaturated fatty acids in them, while animal fats are denser, melt at a higher temperature and contain high levels of saturated fatty acids. It is these saturated fatty acids that have been associated with heart disease.

So it makes good sense to use a plant oil for your basic cooking. Sunflower and safflower seed oils are the lightest, and are rich in polyunsaturated fatty acids; corn, sesame, soy and wheatgerm oils are medium weight; while olive oil is heavier and closer to butter or lard. For general purpose cooking, you could switch from corn to safflower or sunflower oils, using the heavier oils for special dishes. Margarine is not the best choice for cooking (except baking) as its properties rapidly change on heating.

Many traditional dishes cannot be properly made without olive oil, lard, or butter, however. Italian and Mexican cuisines, for instance, call for the particular flavor and weight of olive oil; Chinese cooking benefits from soy oil; the French love butter; pork fat is essential for some dishes of the southern United States. So if you do not want to sacrifice your traditional fats and oils, we recommend that you reserve them for flavoring as much as possible, mixing them with lighter oils for cooking, or simply adding a little to the final dish.

In the Third World, fats normally provide no more than fifteen percent of the total diet, most of it in legumes with only small quantities coming from meat, fish and cooking oil. In the West, we consume three times as much per head,[11] due principally to the larger amounts of animal foods, and vast quantities of cakes, pies, cookies and fried foods that we eat, as well as the liberal way we spread our bread with butter, margarine, peanut butter, and the like.

You can reduce both the total amount of fat you eat and the proportion of saturated fats by cutting down on cakes, pies, cookies and pastries, especially those from the supermarket, which are generally made with heavy fats.

As for spreads, flexible variety is probably more sensible than a hard line. The evidence as to whether butter or margarine is best remains inconclusive. If you like butter, mix it with margarine, or limit it to certain days of the week. You can even make your own margarine by mixing equal quantities of butter and (preferably unrefined) corn or safflower oil. As a change, peanut butter, sesame butter (tahina), sunflower seed butter, and yeast extract are all good spreads. Bread topped with sesame butter and soy bean paste (miso) is one of the contributions of Zen macrobiotics to the western diet.[12] It contains less fat and a broader balance of nutrients than butter or margarine. For a sweeter spread of this kind, try a mixture of sesame butter and honey, known as *halva*.

Guidelines for a balanced diet

GUIDELINE 5 Keep highly processed foods to a minimum

In our view, fresh foods are undoubtedly better than refined and highly processed foods. They have superior taste, texture, and nutritional value. In simple terms, this means that wholewheat bread is preferable to white bread, fresh meat better than hot-dogs and hamburgers, and freshly cooked potatoes, prepared with milk and butter or margarine, better than instant dehydrated mashed potatoes. At breakfast, a homemade wholegrain granola or muesli is better than any of the refined breakfast cereals. Fresh and dried fruits, nuts, and seeds or a freshly baked pie make canned fruit, sugary tarts and frozen puddings seem rather boring and much too sweet. Your chances of good health – physical *and* mental – are certainly increased if you adopt whole fresh foods as your basic diet.

And yet, for thousands of years, people have been salting, smoking, drying, pickling and curing their fresh foods to provide for the winter months when little else is available. Our inheritance of salted herrings, pickles, smoked hams and mackerel, sausages, dried mushrooms and apricots, canned peaches and fruit preserves is a rich one, too rich to throw overboard altogether, even if we can get fresh foods throughout the year now. So if you like your traditional pickles and preserves, don't worry. But if you tend to eat a lot of them, pregnancy would be a good time to cut right down!

Frozen foods can also have an important place in your diet, not only because of their convenience but also because some are actually more nutritious than 'fresh' foods. Vegetables frozen on the farm, for example, sometimes have a higher vitamin content than those that have been stored for long periods before being sold in grocery stores.

Sugar and salt

By eating a lot of refined and processed foods, you will almost certainly be taking in a lot of salt and sugar. In moderation, salt is essential to the diet, and in small quantities sugar is pleasant and harmless. But in excess, both are harmful. Salt is an essential ingredient in the diet, but too much can make you feel tense and at the same time may well raise your blood pressure. Because salt draws water, it can also lead to fluid retention in the body, especially in pregnancy. If you suspect you eat too much salt, experiment with some alternative seasonings: a squeeze of fresh lemon juice, freshly ground pepper, fresh parsley, basil or thyme, or mustard; a spoonful of yogurt, or sesame salt, made from 12–15 parts of sesame seeds roasted in a little oil and crushed into 1 part of coarse sea salt.

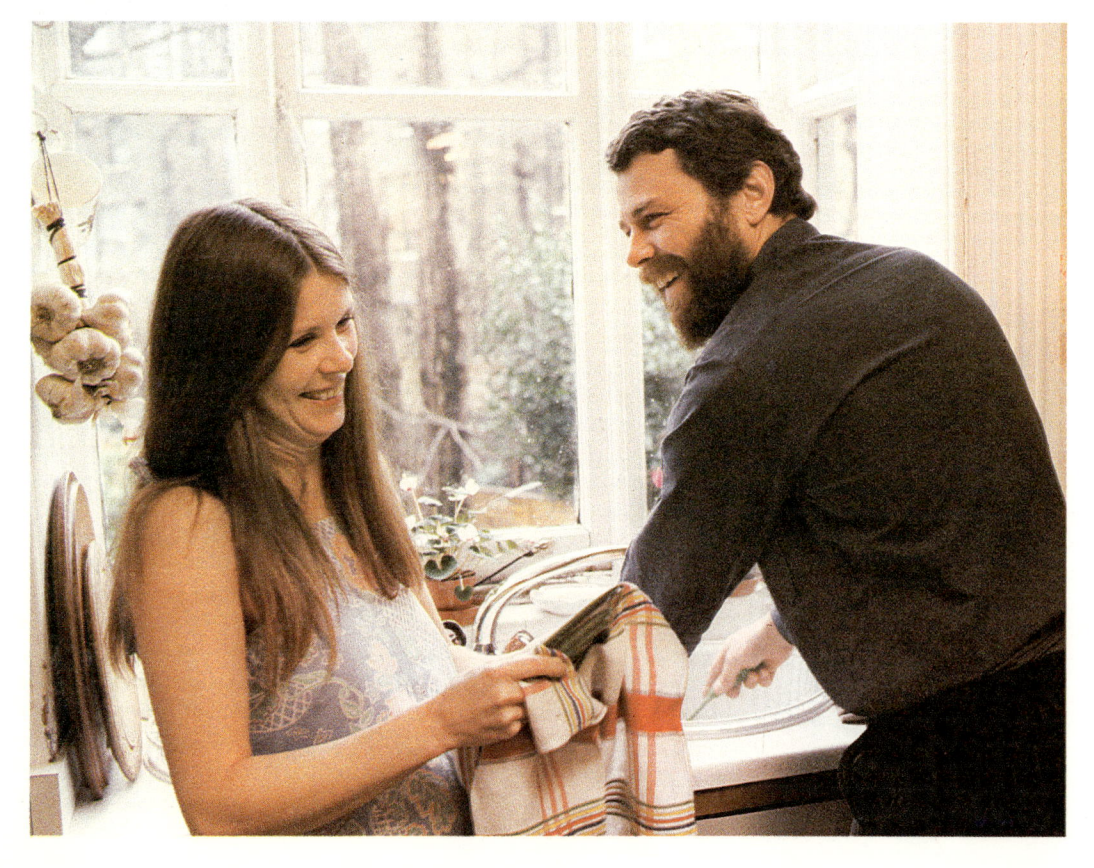

The relationship of the parents is the foundation of the family. Nourishing your baby-to-be with good feelings is as important as a healthy and well-balanced diet.

Guidelines for a balanced diet

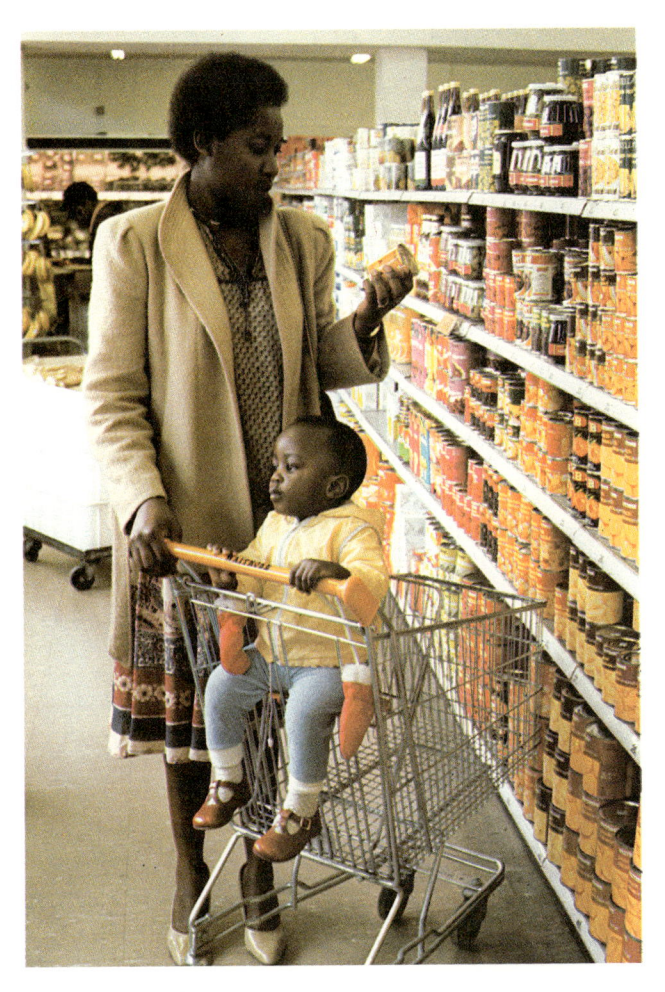

Nobody knows the long-term effects of additives, so try to choose fresh foods whenever possible.

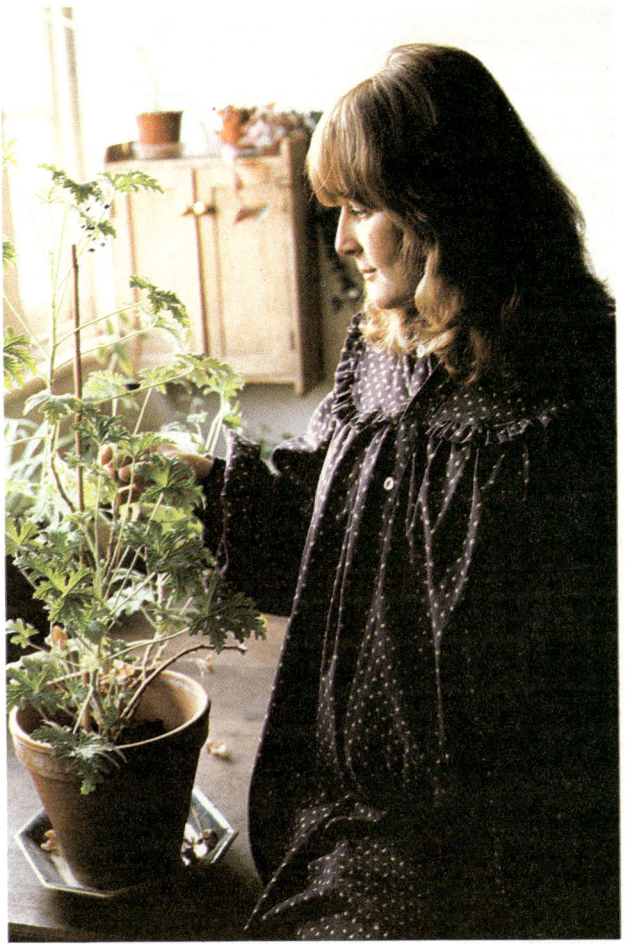

There are many herbs and spices we can grow to add to the flavor of our foods.

Sugar – 'pure, white and deadly' as Professor John Yudkin has called it[13] – was once a sign of affluence, and in many Third World countries it still is. Nor is there any doubt that sugar has made possible a wide range of utterly delicious foods. But eaten in large quantities, it is a major health hazard,[14] implicated in the development of a number of serious degenerative diseases, among them heart disease and diabetes. Sugar is dangerous not only because it is stripped of all the vitamins and minerals that were in the original sugarcane or sugarbeet, but also because it is addictive: it makes you want to eat more and more, thus drawing the appetite away from other, more nourishing foods. In the West, we eat on the average as much as two pounds of sugar each week, a hundred times more than our great-grandparents. The problem is, of course, that we are so often not aware of just how much sugar we are taking in. It comes in many disguises, and is often an added constituent of highly processed foods, too. We consume it in tea, coffee, soft drinks, jams, ice cream, cakes, cookies, and candy, as well as in many canned foods.[13]

Instead of sweets and chocolates, opt for fresh fruits whenever possible. Savor a slice of chilled melon, a bowl of raspberries, or a baked apple: or dip into a mixture of nuts, seeds, and dried fruits. If you are truly addicted to sugar, these foods may not satisfy your cravings at first, but in time they could. Many people find it easier to give up sugar slowly, as sudden withdrawal can sometimes lead to sugar binges. But experiences differ: others (in common with many ex-alcoholics and ex-smokers) say that they were only able to cut down on eating sweet things by giving up the habit altogether. If you have reached the conclusion that sugar must no longer take such a prominent place in your diet, you will have to give careful thought to reducing your intake.

Food additives

Food additives are chemicals added to a product to keep it fresh, to enhance its flavor, to give it a brighter color and to maintain its texture between the factory and the consumer. Synthetic nutrients may also be added to replace a part of those that are lost in the process of refinement. Look carefully at the listings on packs and cans. You will probably be amazed at how long they are.

By law in most western countries, the use of additives is supposed to be strictly controlled. In the words of the United Kingdom Food and Drugs Act, they must be demonstrated as 'necessary and safe'.[15] In practice, the necessity for additives is not always well demonstrated. For example, the thirty permitted additives for use in American bread, and the twenty-four permitted in British bread, are doubtless of economic value to the manufacturers: but whether they are necessary from the consumer's point of view is open to question.

Nor is the safety of the several thousand additives permitted for use always well established. Though many are subject to laboratory testing to see if they harm animals, their activity in the human body – not only individually (as they are tested in the laboratory) but also in combinations (as they are added to food) – is almost impossible to define. It may be that certain combinations of additives are more potent in the body than they are as individual chemicals. In addition, allergy to food additives is now a recognized clinical condition.

The trouble is that testing food additives is a very expensive business.[16] It has been suggested that any manufacturer wishing to use a new additive should pay the cost of adequate testing or not use it.[17] The manufacturers, however, point out that this cost would inevitably be passed on to the consumer, resulting in far higher prices. In the meantime, although public agencies throughout the West work towards the establishment of 'permitted lists' of food additives of all kinds, we and our children will remain the guinea pigs over the long term.

It is also likely that some additives cross the placenta and enter the fetal blood during pregnancy – although to what degree, and with what effect, is hard to say. In rats, the nitrites used to flavor cured meats and ham cross the placenta and at very high doses cause fetal cancer.[18] We cannot extrapolate from this to the human situation but we can note the potential risks. As we eat on average an astonishing two pounds of additives each year, the cumulative effects during pregnancy should be a cause for concern.[19] To minimize your participation in the additive experiment, and to maximize the nutritional value of your diet, we recommend that pregnant women cut down on all refined and factory-processed foods as far as possible.

Chemicals on the farm

Quite apart from the chemicals added intentionally to our food, a number of others are there unintentionally: residues of fertilizers applied to the soil, of pesticides sprayed onto crops, of drugs given to farm animals to maintain their health and growth, as well as the lead from exhaust fumes that settles on the soil. But they are hard to avoid. The entire ecosystem of life on earth is permeated with chemicals. And the effects upon us, at the levels that are commonly reported, remain a question of great controversy.

As many of these chemicals build up in fatty tissue, it is sometimes suggested that we cut all the fat off meat before eating it. We have also been warned to avoid river and lake fish which tend to have higher concentrations of pesticide residues than ocean fish.[20] However, it should be pointed out that ocean fish can also be affected by pollution, especially around coastal areas where industrial activity is high.

Organically grown foods may contain a smaller range of chemical residues, but they are only available to a few. For the vast majority, the effects of chemicals – and the health of our unborn children – are matters for deep concern.

GUIDELINE 6 Take your time!

Compare our guidelines with what you normally eat. If you are enjoying a balanced diet already, you will feel little need to change. But if change does seem to be required, set to it; but take your time. Balance is not found through forced, frantic change. In fact, the process is not unlike weaning. When new foods are gradually introduced into the baby's diet, milk takes a smaller and smaller place: now, during pregnancy, it is your old unbalanced diet that should gradually disappear. Some days, you may find yourself making good progress; on other days (when you feel low, perhaps) the old familiar foods will seem more attractive and you may not be able to resist them very readily. Allow yourself to progress but also to regress a little at times, if you really feel like it: that way, you will make slower but steadier progress than if you push too hard.

Be kind to your blood sugar levels, too, for stress and sudden bursts of intense activity can play havoc with the delicate balance of glucose in the blood. Glucose is needed continually by our muscles for energy, so the blood level has to be maintained within a fine range.

Healthy regulation of the blood sugar level depends on many factors, but two are especially

Guidelines for a balanced diet

important. The first is the way in which our cells burn up glucose for energy. Sudden bursts of activity call for a raised flow of glucose out of the blood and into the muscles. Emotional stresses also increase sugar and oxygen requirements, as does the use of stimulants like coffee and alcohol. Normally, the liver and muscles can supply glucose at short notice, for they contain small stores: but prolonged stress, intense activity and excessive intake of stimulants can set up wide fluctuations in our blood sugar level and gradually undermine its regulation.[21] To maintain a balanced range of blood sugar levels, try to avoid unnecessary stress, cut down on your consumption of stimulants, and get plenty of fresh air.

A second vital influence on the regulation of blood sugar levels is of course the diet, and especially the kind of carbohydrate you eat. Starchy foods like grains, bread, potatoes, bananas and yams are relatively slowly absorbed, and so tend to increase the blood sugar level only very gradually after a meal, while sugary foods – such as sugar itself and sweet cakes or cookies – are absorbed very quickly and tend to raise the blood sugar level rapidly. Any sudden rise calls for rapid adaptation by the rest of the blood sugar regulating system. The pancreas, for example, is required to secrete large quantities of the hormone *insulin*, which directs glucose out of the blood and into body tissue. It is exactly this insulin-producing response of the pancreas that breaks down in the sugar disease *diabetes mellitus*, so that the body is not able to turn all its fuel to best advantage: and there is evidence that eating a lot of sugar is one of its contributory causes.[14,22]

The spirit in which you buy, prepare, and eat your food is also important. For inspiration, go out and buy yourself a new cookbook: and from now on, before you go grocery shopping, take an extra five minutes to reflect on the week's menu. Allow yourself to be enthusiastic about preparing new and nourishing dishes. Take your time and enjoy the preparation of meals. The chances are that if you do so, you will find them both very much more delicious and far more nutritious. Though science could hardly test the hypothesis, we believe that food prepared with pleasure provides far more nourishment than that served up merely out of duty.

Try to avoid the tyranny of mealtimes, too. Regular meals are all very well if they correspond to your rhythms of hunger, but they can also be a bore. Eat when you are hungry – as often as it may be – and stop when you have had enough. This may have its more trying moments when you are under pressure from someone else to eat when you do not feel like it. But if you can maintain your resolve to eat sensibly, others will come to respect your decisions. A pregnant woman is sometimes excused, if she shows a particular fancy for certain types of foods or a determined dietary resolve to avoid certain foodstuffs, where others would perhaps not be.

When it comes to eating, take your time here, too. Chew and savor your food, enjoy its taste and texture. The longer you chew, the less likely you are to overeat or to suffer from indigestion, and the more thoroughly you can break down the food in your mouth before swallowing. Your health can only benefit.

Meanwhile, if you have the occasional urge to buy convenience or fast foods like French fries with ketchup or doughnuts layered with chocolate frosting, don't feel too guilty about it. Just do it, and with pleasure! It will do you no harm, as long as it *is* just the occasional urge and not the start of a binge.

A good cookbook

If wholefoods are relatively new to you, we suggest you buy yourself a new cookbook. During the next twenty years, you are likely to be making up to 20,000 meals for your child, not to mention other members of the family. The right cookbook could make all the difference as to how much you will enjoy the experience, and how well your family turns out to be fed.

Choose carefully. For sound nutrition, steer a middle course between haute cuisine and Zen macrobiotics. Although both have much to commend them, neither gives enough attention to healthy physiology *and* sensual gastronomy. If you have previously paid little attention to recipes, make sure your book is also utterly clear: many cookbook writers take a lot for granted. Any writer who can provide simple ways to combine whole fresh foods in a loving, efficient way will serve you well. If the book turns you on to cooking, and you feel positive about what you are doing, your food will taste better and in turn do you more good. You will find a list of suggested titles on page 91, but you are bound to discover your own favorites, too. Now is also a good time to start collecting recipes from family and friends.

The power of the cook is often underestimated. Yet whoever selects the ingredients and prepares the dish has the chance to effect, most profoundly, the lives of those who sit down to eat it. The cook can delight or depress the family as she wishes. Introduce new recipes now and you will not only refresh your own diet, but your unborn baby's diet, too. Later on, you will have so much else to think about as you begin to care for the new baby, as well as coping with other household tasks, that cooking and the basics of sound nutrition will need to be second nature.

Taboos and temptations

Many great religions contain dietary systems with specific rules as to what may and may not be eaten, both in everyday life and in particular situations such as pregnancy and lactation.[1] Those who observe traditional religious dietary rules are sometimes encouraged to follow other, more 'scientific' principles of nutrition on the assumption that science knows best. In some cases, 'scientific' advice can be very helpful, but in general we recommend anyone who feels positive about their religious food laws to maintain them.

Muslims and Jews, for example, are forbidden to eat blood, and all flesh is supposed to be soaked and drained before cooking. To these peoples, pork is also taboo. On the other hand, some societies have thrived on the pig, and still do. Navajo Indians are forbidden to eat fish or wild turkey, Hindus may not eat the holy cow, while Brahmans do not eat any meat at all. For other reasons, perhaps, a high proportion of adult Africans, American Indians, and oriental peoples do not drink milk, and indeed lack the enzymes to digest it properly.

Members of these various ethnic groups debate among themselves the origin and importance of their rules, with any number of scientific and pseudo-scientific arguments being thrown in for good measure. Yet it may well be that we in the West can learn from their ancient wisdom.

In South and Central America, in China, Malaya and the Philippines, in Pakistan and the Sahara, there has been for thousands of years a system by which all foods are known not by their chemical composition but by their relative qualities in producing heat or cold in the body. According to these systems, pregnancy – a condition in which energy accumulates in the body – is a 'hot' state and so calls for a diet of cold foods. Very hot foods are considered dangerous. In southern India, for example, papaya – a tropical fruit – is considered hot and believed to create a risk of uterine bleeding.[2,3] This may be because it is rich in Vitamin C, which has been used, in large doses, to stimulate abortion very early in pregnancy.[4] The hot/cold systems of nutrition – including the Chinese yin/yang system on which Zen macrobiotics is based – display an impressive uniformity throughout certain areas of the world.

More 'magical' pregnancy taboos have also been reported. One South American tribe, for example, prohibits eating the meat of a local spotted rodent because it is said to give a baby spots; another – in West Africa – will not permit a pregnant woman to eat squirrel meat. These creatures shelter in the holes of trees and it is believed that any fetus nourished by such an animal might be tempted to hide too long in the womb and create a difficult birth.[5]

If you grew up subject to special food laws, consider them well before throwing them out: they may have served your people for centuries – perhaps in unexpected ways – and they may do the same for you. If you find yourself in serious doubt about what you eat, however, and think you may need dietary advice, consult your doctor.

Alcohol and caffeine

What you *drink* has just as much of an effect on your body as what you *eat* and – as with our guidelines on food – we recommend that you follow your own intuition as to what you drink, but within certain limits. Alcohol, tea, coffee, cocoa, and sweetened soft drinks can all, if drunk to excess, harm the fetus: so do keep them to a minimum.

Most adults are affected to some degree by half an ounce of pure ethanol, which is the amount of alcohol in a glass of wine or two cans of light beer. Animal experiments suggest that drinking *three times* this amount each day increases the risk of congenital abnormality,[6] and that even smaller amounts can temporarily affect the fetal nervous system.[7] In humans, there is less evidence: only chronic alcoholism has been associated with congenital abnormality – though one case has been reported of abnormality following a single massive alcohol binge in the early weeks of pregnancy.[8] However, alcoholics also tend to smoke and to eat poorly (alcohol is biochemically a refined carbohydrate, which may take the place of other more nourishing foods in the diet), so the harm done by alcohol alone is not clear.

There is no firmly-established 'safe dose', though one or two glasses of wine or beer a day, or a single spirit, is generally recognized as safe.[9] It should be pointed out, however, that for some women, perhaps those unfamiliar with alcohol consumption, even a relatively low level of alcohol intake may be too much and therefore harmful.[10,11]

Alcoholism is generally associated with vitamin and mineral depletion, notably of Vitamins C, B_1, B_2, and folic acid. If you have been a heavy drinker, you should probably be taking low-level supplements during your pregnancy.

Coffee, tea, and cocoa, as well as carbonated drinks made from the cola plant, all contain the stimulant *caffeine*, which alters both the blood chemistry and nutrient requirements. These also need to be treated with caution. Some studies suggest that moderate caffeine intake in pregnancy is safe;[12,13] although one, by the American physician Lechtat, gives the impression that even low levels may be harmful for some women.[14] At high levels, however, caffeine can be poisonous. An increased incidence of low birth-weight babies has been found in women who drink more than seven cups of coffee a day, and this risk is increased if freshly brewed coffee is used. As you can see from the table, the caffeine content of different coffee preparations, as well as that of tea and cocoa, varies considerably. Five hundred milligrams of caffeine per day is probably a safe maximum for most women.

Caffeine in beverages and food

Coffee, brewed fresh	75–150 mg./8 ounce cup
Coffee, instant	30–80 mg./8 ounce cup
Tea	40–50 mg./8 ounce cup
Cola	20–40 mg./8 ounce cup
Cocoa	2–40 mg./8 ounce cup
Milk chocolate	12 mg./2 ounce bar

Many pregnant women actually feel repulsed by alcohol, tea, and coffee, almost as if their bodies were warning them of possible ill-effects. If this happens to you, welcome the change. You might try herbal teas instead. They can be surprisingly refreshing. Peppermint and camomile are mild natural tranquilizers that have been recommended for morning sickness and indigestion. Red raspberry leaf tea and spikenard have for centuries been used during late pregnancy to promote a relaxed delivery.[15] A sachet or a handful of leaves infused for five minutes is all you need.

Fresh fruit and vegetable juices are also good beverages, while milk in moderation is nourishing – though in the large quantities at times recommended for pregnancy, in some it can cause nasal congestion, running colds or eczema. Avoid sweetened fruit-flavored juices and soft drinks. They are usually of little nutritional value, contain more additives than other drinks, and take the place of more beneficial beverages.

Smoking

Despite the fact that smoking is a well-publicized threat to pregnancy, tobacco remains the commonest addictive drug used by pregnant women. Encouraged by over 100 million dollars worth of advertising each year, tobacco sales to pregnant women remain high, especially to teenagers and low-income women.[16]

Although tobacco smoke contains a number of potentially harmful toxins, the effects in pregnancy are not always apparent. In general, healthy, young first-time mothers who are light smokers show little ill-effect; but the older a woman becomes, the more children she has had, and the more she smokes, the greater are the risks of impaired fetal growth, and spontaneous abortion.[17,18] Under a microscope, the blood vessels of a heavy smoker's placenta are prematurely 'aged', while her blood usually contains abnormally low levels of Vitamins B_{12}, C and folic acid.[19]

Fresh coffee can be delicious: but it is also a potent stimulant. Pregnancy is the ideal time for you to explore alternatives, like herb teas or hot lemon and honey.

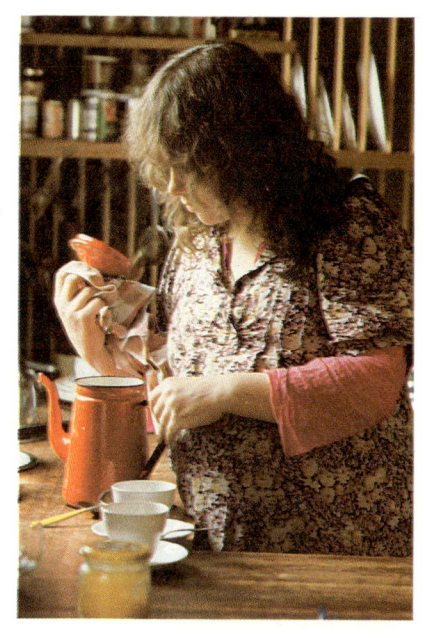

However, the exact effect of tobacco is hard to define: smokers tend to be poorer, live under more stress, and drink more alcohol and caffeine than non-smokers. They are also more likely to be working out of the house and are less likely to be attending pre-natal clinics.[20,21] As all these adverse living conditions can retard fetal growth, it is clear, as Professor Yerushalmy of the University of Jerusalem has pointed out, that "even before these women started to smoke, they were destined to have smaller babies".[22]

Yet, odd though it may seem, smoking actually appears to serve a useful purpose for some women. For the effects of tobacco can be hypotensive, which means that smoking calms some women and reduces their blood pressure by dilating the size of the blood vessels. In pregnancy, one of the effects of this is to reduce the rate of toxemia among smokers. Induction of labor and forceps deliveries are also less likely to occur with smokers.[23,24] However, for heavy smokers who do develop toxemia, the chances of serious complications at birth are very high.[25]

But it is not always easy to stop smoking, especially for women, as one recent review has shown.[26,27] For those who cannot stop, pregnancy can become a nightmare of guilt and anxiety: and no one can say what damage this may do to the pregnancy.[28] Those who do manage to stop smoking sometimes turn to sweets instead: others maintain their self-control only at the price of great mental stress. For these women, it may be more sensible to smoke the occasional guilt-free cigarette and thereby avoid excessive tension. We do *not* recommend smoking, but we do feel it important to be realistic.

The nutrients in pregnancy

Nutrients are the chemical components of our food, the stuff of which the plants and animals we eat are made. They are also the very stuff of which our bodies are made and are in a constant state of action and reaction, their relationships changing with every breath we take. The fantastic, harmonious complexity of these changing relationships is maintained by a self-ordering system known as *metabolism*.

All our physical and mental activities take place by virtue of metabolism. This includes the processes whereby food, water and air are taken into our bodies and transformed there into living tissue – in pregnancy, both your tissue and the baby's – and into energy for daily life.

The nutrients are classified into six chemical groups: *carbohydrates*, *fats* and *proteins* (*macro-nutrients*) which we need in fairly large quantities to supply us with energy and to maintain our body tissues; *fiber*, which may also be considered as a macro-nutrient because we need quite a lot of it for healthy digestion; and *vitamins* and *minerals* (the *micro-nutrients*) that provide small but vital amounts of materials not only for our body tissues but also for the enzymes and hormones that regulate our metabolism.

The carbohydrates

This group of nutrients provides our main source of energy, fueling the fires of metabolism. Most dietary carbohydrate comes from grains, bananas, and starchy root vegetables like potatoes and yams. In the western world, sugar is also an important source. The carbohydrate from grains is *starch*, which appears under the microscope as long chains of glucose and other similar small molecules, while the carbohydrate in sugar appears as simple glucose molecules.

Most of the carbohydrate we eat is broken down into glucose in the small intestine before being absorbed into the blood. After a carbohydrate meal, the concentration of glucose in the blood (the blood sugar level) is raised. At the same time, however, glucose is being taken out of the blood for use as energy by the muscles, the brain, and the body's internal organs. This flow of glucose in and out of the blood is among the most complex and finely controlled mechanisms in the body, and in healthy people it ensures that the blood sugar level remains within a particular range.

The amount of carbohydrate delivered to the fetus – who also needs it for energy – will depend upon the amount of glucose and oxygen in the mother's blood. Early in pregnancy, the placenta will have set up carbohydrate stores to protect the fetus against any temporary shortage. Later on, the fetus will lay down his own carbohydrate store in the liver, as the enzymes that carry out the reactions involved develop.[1]

These fetal stores will provide your baby with a source of instant energy both during and after the birth. Babies born prematurely, however, before these stores have been set up, quickly become glucose-depleted. Low birth-weight babies, and those who have had a traumatic, energy-depleting delivery, even if they are fully grown, also tend to become glucose-depleted: and for these babies, sugar water is often required soon after delivery.

The proteins

The structure of every living cell is made largely of protein: so are the hormones and the many forms of chemical carrier that transport nutrients around the body. Antibodies, which protect us from certain kinds of infection, are also largely made of protein.

All proteins are made up of smaller units called *amino acids*. Of the twenty-three known amino acids, our bodies can make fifteen (babies, only fourteen) but the remainder need to be obtained from food and are called *essential amino acids*. The proteins in animal foods – meat, fish, eggs and dairy products – contain all eight essential amino acids and are known as *complete proteins*. Plant proteins – those in grains, legumes and many kinds of nut – lack one essential amino acid and so are called *incomplete proteins*. As grains, legumes and nuts each lack a different amino acid, a combination of grains and legumes, or grains and nuts, makes a complete protein.

You do need extra protein in pregnancy, but not as much as you might think. Protein deficiency is rare in western society. But in the Third World, where severe, prolonged food shortage is relatively common in pregnancy, it is associated with low birth-weight, under-developed babies. Here and in other low income groups, additional protein in pregnancy is beneficial: an extra serving of maize and beans may be all that is needed. In those countries where 'more' has come to mean 'better', a substantial increase in protein intake is commonly recommended. Yet a high protein diet may in fact be harmful. Several studies have demonstrated this. The most recent were undertaken in New York in the 1970s. Dr H.J. Osofsky at the Temple University Hospital supplemented the diet of 122 women with high protein and mineral supplements, and found a significant decrease in the babies' birth weight and physical coordination compared with a control group.[2] These results were confirmed by Professor David Rush at the Albert Einstein College of Medicine, who reported that mothers taking a high protein supplement gave birth to lighter babies. Rush did find, however, that a balanced, moderate-protein supplement can reduce the risk of low birth weight.[3]

This is confirmed by the long-term experience of the Montreal Diet Dispensary in Canada, where a supplement of milk, eggs and oranges given free to needy mothers has been shown to reduce the low birth weight figures.[4] Such studies confirm our experience that it is more sensible to balance your overall diet, without particular emphasis on any one nutrient (unless your doctor has confirmed special requirements in *your* particular case), increasing your general food intake according to hunger.

Your developing baby needs protein both to build up his body tissue and to develop a store of antibodies to disease. For his tissue, the protein is thought to be built up from amino acids that cross the placenta. Immunity proteins, called *immunoglobulins*, seem to cross whole, from the mother's blood to the baby's. In this way, your full-term newborn will already have acquired resistance to certain diseases to which you are resistant.

The fats

Fat is required both to maintain the healthy structure of our body cells and as a source of energy when carbohydrate is scarce. It comes in many forms from both the animal and the plant world, giving our food a broad variety of textures and tastes. A fat-free diet – without any oils, butter, sauces, nuts, seeds, or fatty fish or meat – becomes terribly monotonous. Nevertheless, we can survive for long periods with very little dietary fat. Composed of smaller units called *fatty acids*, most of this group of nutrients can be manufactured in our bodies from carbohydrates: but two fatty acids can be obtained only from our diet. These are the *essential fatty acids*: safflower and sunflower seed oils are a good source.

In the past ten years, the types of fat we eat have been given immense publicity. Strong links have been identified between a diet rich in meat fats, butter, and cream – that is, those fats rich in saturated fatty acids – and a number of diseases, especially heart disease. The amount of *cholesterol* (a fat-carbohydrate molecule) in our diet also appears to be directly linked with heart disease. Yet a certain amount of saturated fat and cholesterol in the diet may also be essential, and the evidence linking these substances with heart disease is not conclusive. This is in fact a highly controversial area of nutrition. In Japan, for example, fat consumption is relatively low, yet the incidence of strokes is much higher than in the West. In the United States, a recent decline in the amounts of saturated fatty acids and cholesterol in the diet has been linked with lower rates of stroke and coronary heart disease: but the evidence has been strongly challenged, for the stroke rate has actually been declining for at least twenty-five years, much longer than the trend towards a reduction in animal fats and butter.[5]

In view of this uncertainty, it does seem sensible to cut down on animal foods. Do your basic cooking with corn and sunflower oils, which are rich in unsaturated fatty acids: and try snacking on sunflower seeds and nuts instead of cookies or bread with butter. Sunflower seeds are rich in polyunsaturated fatty acids, which are reported to reverse the thickening of the artery walls in *atherosclerosis*.[6] They are also delicious.

During the early part of pregnancy, most mothers lay down a store of fat weighing 6–8 lbs – mostly in the thighs – which is widely believed to be an energy reserve in preparation for breastfeeding after the birth. Only during the last month of pregnancy does fat also pass in substantial amounts to the fetus, so that a full-term baby has sufficient to provide him with energy for the first 48 hours after delivery, a period during which most newborn babies drink very little milk.[7] Premature and low–birth–weight babies, however, have very small fat stores and so need earlier feeding.

Fiber

Fiber – or roughage – is found in the bran of grains, in starchy root vegetables, in fruits, and in the coats of seeds, nuts and legumes. Without it, the intestines become congested, so that constipation results: and over a period of years, fiber deficiency may cause *diverticulitis* and other diseases of the digestive tract, hemorrhoids, and varicose veins. Fiber can also reduce abnormally high cholesterol levels in the blood. A balanced diet of fresh, whole foods will ensure that you get plenty of fiber. The table shows that there are many good sources. There should be no need to take extra bran.

SOURCES OF DIETARY FIBER

Bread	Vegetables	Fruits
Cornbread	All raw vegetables	Apples with skin
Crackers with seeds	Brussels sprouts	Berries
	Cabbage	Dried apricots
Pumpernickel	Corn	Pears with skin
Rye bread	Parsnips	Prunes
Rye crisp bread	Peas	Raisins
Wholegrain crackers	**Nuts and seeds**	**Cereals**
Wholemeal bread	**Legumes**	Bran
Grains	Baked beans	Oatmeal
Brown rice	Black-eyed peas	
Buckwheat	Chickpeas	
Wheat germ	Kidney beans	
	Lima beans	

The micro-nutrients in pregnancy

Vitamins are tiny substances obtained from plants and animals that our bodies need but that we cannot (at least, in theory) make for ourselves. In practice, a number of vitamins *can* be made in our bodies: Vitamin D, for example, is made in the skin on the action of sunlight. Less than a century ago, none but a few inspired scientists guessed that vitamins even existed, while the very idea that a diet deficient in such unproven substances could cause disease was a heresy. Today we know better, but we are still far from the complete story. Thirteen vitamins have so far been identified and widely accepted by the scientific community. The list is likely to grow. And vitamin deficiency is now, of course, a well-recognized cause of disease.

Vitamin deficiency during pregnancy can also harm the fetus, although the exact nature of the risks is hard to assess. From animal experiments, we know that a lack of many individual nutrients from the diet can cause specific abnormalities, depending on the stage of pregnancy reached at the time of deficiency. In humans, there is much less specific information because of the ethical objection to researching on mothers. But there is, for example, some evidence that *spina bifida*, a defect of the central nervous system, is caused by vitamin deficiency in pregnancy.[1,2] In 1982, the British Medical Research Council initiated a five-year study of the effects of vitamin supplements (and especially folic acid) on women at risk of delivering spina bifida babies to test the hypothesis.[3]

Other vitamin deficiencies in pregnancy are known to affect the baby. Severely inadequate intakes of Vitamins A, B_1, B_6 and folic acid have all been reported in mothers and their newborn babies.[4] A severe lack of B_1, for example, which comes from eating a lot of white rice or white bread and not enough B_1-rich foods like whole grains, legumes, seeds, meat and fish – has long been known to cause *beriberi* – a disease of the nerves and muscles – in both mother and baby. And Vitamin B_6 deficiency in mothers has been associated with poor muscle tone and reduced respiration at birth in their babies.[5] Rich sources of Vitamin B_6 include herring, salmon, liver, yeast, nuts, brown rice, wheat germ and blackstrap molasses.

Vitamin D deficiency in pregnancy seems largely confined to dark-skinned women living in sun-starved inner cities.[6] For Vitamin D is synthesized in our skin when the sun shines on it, and dark-skinned ethnic groups – who are generally accustomed to a lot of sun – easily become deficient in a cloudy environment. If they do not eat foods containing Vitamin D, like herring, salmon, pilchards, sardines, eggs, or cod-liver oil, their babies have a tendency towards low birth weight and disturbance of calcium metabolism (which is regulated by Vitamin D), with nervous and skeletal abnormalities.

Although many popular writers give the impression that these, and a good many other vitamin deficiencies, are common in pregnancy, the truth is that no one really knows. Marginal vitamin intake (not severe deficiency but not optimal intake either) has been reported to be relatively common in the West,[7] although the criteria for deciding what is adequate and what is not vary from one researcher to the next; and most western public health authorities have, during the early 1980s, recommended major dietary changes with a view to increasing vitamin intake among a number of other objectives. But it is almost impossible to say quite what proportion of the population is truly vitamin-deficient and in what respects.

If, according to our guidelines, you feel that your diet over recent years has been poor, or if you think you may have become vitamin-depleted through previous pregnancies or prolonged drug use (including the contraceptive pill), then extra vitamins may be a good idea for you. And if you are a vegetarian, don't forget that you need a source of Vitamin B_{12} both during your pregnancy and after the birth. If you want to know more precisely what *you* need, you should consult a nutritionist, who can assess your diet to see if, theoretically, you are getting what you need. Hair or blood analysis is also used by some physicians to identify possible deficiencies, but such analysis is expensive and not always reliable. For this reason, low level supplements of vitamins (about ten times the recommended daily allowance) are sometimes prescribed without analysis. This is a matter for you and your doctor to decide.

But if you have eaten well during previous years, and have not been subject to the depleting effect of previous pregnancies or prolonged use of drugs, it is less likely that supplements will help you. This is confirmed by American researchers Hemminki and Starfield at The John Hopkins University in a study of all the properly controlled clinical trials of supplementation in pregnancy they were able to trace.[8] They found no evidence that healthy, well-nourished women benefit from extra vitamins. If, however, you or your doctor consider it best to take low-level supplements, try to find a brand made from natural ingredients (usually from plant extracts). The synthetic vitamins are sometimes poorly absorbed and are therefore not so readily effective.

While low-level supplements (whether necessary or not) are probably harmless, high level megadose supplements (often a hundred times the recommended daily intake) may be harmful in pregnancy. Mothers who take large doses of

Vitamins A or D, for example, are probably putting their babies at risk, though here again it is animal studies that provide the suggestive evidence.[9,10] Your doctor will advise the recommended doses.

Excessive intake of Vitamin C may also be harmful, as animal experiments have shown. Pregnant guinea pigs given doses of 25 milligrams per kilogram of body weight have shorter pregnancies with more risk of stillbirths and premature births.[11,12] This is equivalent to 1.5 grams per day for an adult human. Now, we have known pregnant mothers who insisted on taking this amount (and more) every day without apparent ill effect, but there does seem to be a risk, especially during the first three months after conception. There is one short report of twenty women who wished to terminate their pregnancies and took six grams of Vitamin C each per day, for three days, during this critical period, to see if it brought on 'spontaneous' abortion. For sixteen of them, it did. The report included no clinical details, however, and there was no untreated control group with which to draw a good comparison.

There may be yet another form of risk to the fetus if the mother takes megadoses of Vitamin C. This substance, *ascorbic acid*, readily crosses the placenta and a fetus could become dependent on the high levels he receives through the cord. Vitamin dependency is largely uncharted territory, but there is evidence that regular high doses can cause a physiological adaptation and a need for high doses. The process is not unlike addiction to other drugs: and if the vitamin supplements are suddenly stopped, deficiency readily occurs.

Among adults, this appears to have happened during World War II, when the Vitamin C deficiency disease, *scurvy*, was apparently higher among those who had previously taken Vitamin C supplements.[13] Two more recent cases of scurvy have been reported in otherwise healthy adults who abandoned Vitamin C supplements and returned to a low ascorbic acid diet.[14] As Vitamin C crosses the placenta in pregnancy, it seems likely that babies can become dependent in the womb on their mother's high Vitamin C intake, and then become deficient after the birth if supplements are not continued. One study, by Canadian researcher Dr. W. Cochrane, reports exactly this: scurvy among the infants of mothers who took a lot of Vitamin C during pregnancy.[15] As there is no known advantage to taking more than a gram of Vitamin C per day during pregnancy – despite what the Vitamin C vendors claim – you can safely avoid megadoses without fearing that you are losing out. Five hundred milligrams per day should be an ample amount to take as supplementation during your pregnancy.

Vitamins in common foods

Eat something from each vitamin group every day.

Vitamin	Rich sources
A	Liver, sweet potato, melon, dark green leafy vegetables
B_1	Whole grains, especially the germ and bran ham, kidneys, brewer's yeast
B_2	Liver, kidney, brewer's yeast, meat, and yeast extracts
B_3	Peanuts, bran, liver, kidney, poultry, fish, wheat germ
B_6	Whole grains, especially the germ and bran nuts, fish, liver, molasses
B_{12}	Meat, fish, eggs, cheese
C	Oranges, lemons, currants, cabbage, potatoes, avocado
D	Herrings, mackerel, sardines, cod-liver oil
E	Nuts, seeds, wheat germ and their unprocessed oils
Folic acid	Asparagus, spinach, lentils, beans, bran, liver, yeast

Vitamin	Moderate sources
A	Butter, cheese, cream, eggs, apricots, mango, prunes
B_1	Vegetables and legumes (especially raw), fish, meat, eggs, seeds
B_2	Vegetables, nuts, wheat germ, meat, fish, eggs, cheese
B_3	Dried fruit, potatoes, meat, legumes, cheese, nuts
B_6	Banana, avocado, apricot, meat, vegetables, legumes
C	Corn, liver, kidney, apples, banana, plums, carrots
D	Eggs, butter, cheese, enriched margarine or milk
E	Cabbage, sweet potatoes, bran, apples, banana, currants
Folic acid	Whole grains, mushrooms, egg, dark green leafy vegetables

Minerals are quite literally the particles of rock and earth that are present in foods, and that we and all other living organisms need to eat for our good health. Some – like *calcium* and *phosphorus* – we need in relatively large quantities because they form part of our very flesh and bones. Others – like *iron*, *iodine*, *zinc* and *copper* – we need in relatively small quantities, less than one-ten-thousandth of our body weight, in fact: their functions tend to be metabolic rather than structural. To date, fifteen minerals are known to be essential for human health and, within the 1980s, another five are likely to be widely accepted as vital.[16]

Calcium is perhaps the best known. Together with *phosphorus*, it forms the basis of our bones and teeth. An old wives' tale warns that for every child a woman bears she will lose one tooth, and in poorly nourished women – especially if they have had several babies already – this can indeed occur. For the fetus must have his calcium and will draw what he needs from the mother's bones and teeth if her diet is inadequate.

There is, however, no need for a well-nourished pregnant woman drastically to increase her calcium intake: your appetite, the increased absorption of calcium from your food, and the greater retention of calcium by the kidneys will ensure that you and your baby get what you need.[17] Nor should we underestimate the power of the body to adapt to even very low intakes of calcium. Medical researcher Dr. I. Shenolikar has reported that Indian women, eating only one third of the amount of calcium recommended for pregnant women in the United States, had adapted to the increasing demands of the fetus within three months of becoming pregnant.[18] This appears to be confirmed by the work of Professor A. R. Walker in South Africa who studied the X-rays of Bantu mothers eating an equally low-calcium diet, and found no evidence of skeletal demineralization, even among women with seven or more children.[19]

In the light of this, there is no sense in drinking two pints of milk a day "for the extra calcium and protein", as we are sometimes told, unless you really feel like it. As we have seen, extra protein is of no particular advantage unless your normal diet is low in protein, and the same may well be true of calcium. In addition, some people cannot tolerate milk: a high percentage of adult Blacks, Orientals and American Indians lack the enzymes to digest it. The condition known as *lactose intolerance* leads to abdominal cramps and diarrhea when milk is drunk. This form of cramp is quite different from the calf cramps that occur in some women during pregnancy, often at night. Calcium is widely prescribed as treatment for calf cramps and often appears to be effective, although controlled trials show that the effect of a placebo (without any calcium content at all) is sometimes just as good.[20] Massage and stretching are excellent remedies for most leg cramps, the majority of sufferers find.

There are many sources of calcium. If you really like milk, by all means drink a pint a day, but you can also find calcium in nuts (especially almonds and filberts); seeds, like sesame; dark green leafy vegetables, like kale, cabbage, and parsley; small fish eaten with their bones, like sardines and pilchards; eggs and cheese; and molasses. Brewer's yeast is another good source. Wholemeal bread contains moderate amounts of calcium: but for those who are used to white bread, absorption of the wholewheat calcium is low at first. It may take up to three months of eating wholewheat bread for the development in your intestine of the enzymes required to release the calcium.[19]

The need for iron

Iron is the most controversial mineral in pregnancy nutrition. Although routinely prescribed by most physicians from the third month, it is probably needed only by less than one out of every ten women. And for some, iron supplements can have unpleasant side-effects.

Iron's main function in our body is within the red blood cells, where it forms part of the hemoglobin molecule. *Hemoglobin* enables the blood to carry oxygen from the lungs to other cells of the body, where it plays a vital part in energy production. One of the signs of iron-deficiency anemia is thus a lack of energy. Iron also makes the blood red, so that another sign of deficiency is a very pale skin color.

In pregnancy, your need for iron increases as your blood volume increases, but this additional requirement is normally satisfied by a number of adaptations that occur quite naturally. Menstruation stops and with it, iron losses in the blood (although there may be losses later, during labor). Secondly, absorption of iron from food increases in pregnancy, by anything from two to tenfold,[21] as it does for other nutrients. In fact, there is some evidence that the less iron there *is* in your diet, the greater the absorption.[22]

Your hunger will also increase in pregnancy, and the extra food will, if you eat well, give you extra iron. A balanced diet, with plenty of iron-rich foods (not only liver and other meats, but shellfish or legumes like soybeans and kidney beans, sesame and sunflower seeds, and dried fruits – especially apricots) will normally give you all the additional iron you need.

Why, then, are iron supplements routinely prescribed by so many doctors? The reason is that for some women, the adaptations of pregnancy are inadequate to prevent deficiency.[23] A poor diet in the past may have reduced their liver stores of iron, especially if there have been previous nutrient-draining pregnancies. If not already anemic, they may now become so, with a risk of severe anemia later if they lose a lot of blood at the birth. However, one recent Danish study suggests that this is the case for no more than one in ten pregnant women in the West, perhaps more in low-income areas.[24]

If iron deficiency were easy to spot, it would be possible simply to give supplements to those in need. But a lack of energy and paleness can be due to many things; even blood tests may not help the diagnosis. Your doctor will probably take periodic blood samples during the pregnancy in order to check the hemoglobin concentration of your blood, but in fact hemoglobin is a rather poor indicator of the amount of iron in the body: it only shows the concentration of iron in the blood, and nothing of the sometimes considerable stores in the liver and kidneys. Nor is a falling hemoglobin concentration in pregnancy necessarily a sign of iron deficiency, because it tends to fall quite naturally during early pregnancy, leveling off at about 35 weeks.[25] This seems to be because the blood volume increases by about half in pregnancy, while the total amount of hemoglobin only increases by about a quarter: so the actual amount of iron in the blood does not decrease, only the concentration does. Other blood tests for determining a mother's iron status can provide clearer information but they are expensive; so the hemoglobin tests continue: and to guard against any false impressions they may give, most physicians recommend routine iron supplements to protect mothers and their babies against risk of deficiency.

Iron supplements and side-effects

If iron supplements were entirely harmless, there would be no problem with this practice. But many women find them indigestible: they tend to cause constipation and sometimes stomach cramps. There is also evidence that they interfere with the absorption of other nutrients from the intestines – Vitamin E[26] and zinc,[27,28] for example. British researchers D.J. Taylor and T. Lind have pointed to yet another side effect: ten percent of women taking iron tablets tend to develop very large, fragile, short-lived red blood cells.[29]

In 1965, an expert committee of the World Health Organization deplored the indiscriminate issue of iron preparations to all pregnant women.[30] Ten years later, Professor A. M. Thomson, one of the most distinguished infant nutritionists of the century, added that "the effects of giving large doses of extra iron is to increase the red blood cell volume and the number of red blood cells. Whether such a practice is entirely harmless is at least worth questioning. Our practice is NOT to give pregnant women large doses of iron... unless there is evidence that clinical anemia is developing with a hemoglobin concentration of less than 10 grams per deciliter that is falling rapidly".[31]

If you had a good diet before the pregnancy, with plenty of iron-rich foods, and continue with that diet now, you are unlikely to need iron supplements. Good sources include not only meat, especially liver, and shellfish but also legumes like soybeans, kidney beans and lentils; sunflower, sesame and pumpkin seeds; and dark green leafy vegetables (especially spinach and kale).

If you take iron supplements, they are best absorbed if taken immediately before or after a meal, especially if the meal contains meat. Should you feel any reaction, try taking them between meals, when they are less well absorbed but appear to cause fewer side-effects, and see your doctor. Folic acid is frequently prescribed at the same time, as is Vitamin B_{12}.

Minerals in Common Foods

Mineral	Rich sources
Calcium	Nuts, seeds, milk, cheese, eggs, sardines with bones
Phosphorus	Fish, liver, kidneys, nuts, whole grains, cheese, seeds
Iron	Wheat germ, bran, kidneys, liver, shellfish, nuts
Iodine	Seafood, sunflower seeds, cod-liver oil, seaweeds
Zinc	Herrings, oysters, cheese, sunflower seeds, beans
Copper	Seafood, meat, nuts, seeds, soybeans, wheat germ, bran

Mineral	Moderate sources
Calcium	Oats, bran, fish, figs, cocoa, dark green leafy vegetables
Phosphorus	Shellfish, white rice, meat, legumes, mushrooms, dried fruit
Iron	Meat, herring, mackerel, legumes, spinach, dried fruit
Iodine	Liver, eggs, peanuts, pineapple, mayonnaise, iodized salt
Zinc	Grains, legumes, carrots, fish, avocados, peanuts, corn
Copper	Grains, vegetables, eggs, apples, lemons, strawberries

Energy, calories and weight gain

Energy, the force of life on earth, is found locked up in all living organisms, including our food and also our own bodies. During the process of metabolism, potential energy in food is released into dynamic energy-muscle movements and heat inside our body cells, for example. This release of energy is a sort of chemical burning, and oxygen is essential for this reaction, just as it is for any fire. The amount of heat released from any particular food is measured in *calories*. Each gram of protein or carbohydrate absorbed into our bodies carries a potential four calories of energy; each gram of fat carries nine. Vitamins, minerals and fiber contribute negligible amounts of energy.

We need a constant intake of energy to fuel our lives, but the amounts we need vary enormously. Just as our requirements for individual nutrients may vary, so energy requirements are not constant. Among the most important factors that decide what *you* as an individual need are your lean body weight and your normal metabolic rate. Fat people generally have a slow metabolic rate. They burn their food slowly, so that over-eating can easily lead to the excess energy being stored as fat. But if they take more exercise *and* eat less, calories can be lost. Exercise tends to raise the metabolic rate, so that calories are more efficiently burned, whilst eating less also helps to prevent further fat stores being laid down.

As your pregnancy develops, your need for calories will increase, both to provide for the growing fetus and to set up an energy store for breastfeeding after the birth. This means you will feel like eating more, but not necessarily that much more because, in pregnancy, the metabolic rate slows down, which has the effect of conserving energy in the body. On the average, healthy women gain 20–30 pounds during pregnancy – that is, about one half-pound per week for the first six months and one pound per week thereafter – but the range is actually wider than that. We have known perfectly healthy mothers *take off* weight during the first three months (one of them described it as her body finding its right weight) with a net gain of only 10–15 pounds. Dr T. Brewer, in his Californian study, found a natural variation from around zero to over 40 pounds without apparent ill effect.[1]

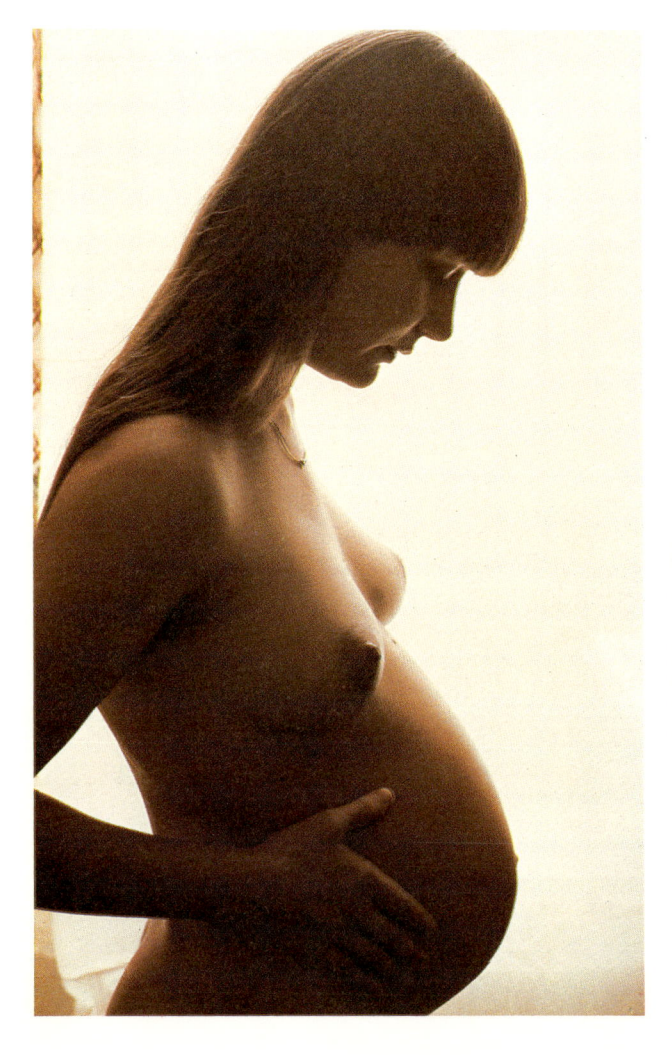

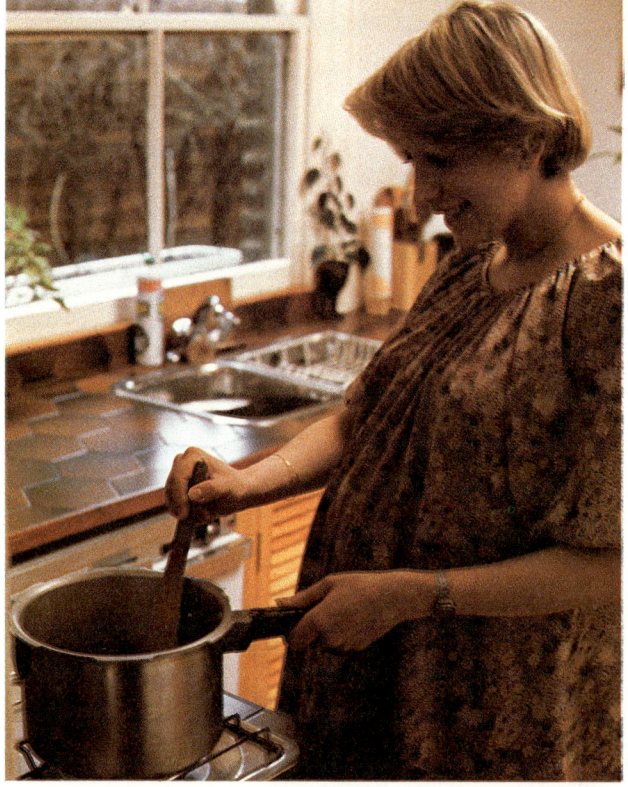

Weighing is one way of checking that all is well: but keeping in touch with your own body can be even more enlightening.

If your diet is balanced and your sense of hunger working well, weight gain will probably be within the average range.

Weight gain and toxemia

For many years, it was believed that a weight gain of over thirty pounds put a pregnant woman at risk of toxemia, but this view is now discredited.[2,3] *Toxemia* is a condition in which the mother has raised blood pressure (*hypertension*), water retention (*edema*) and the excretion of protein in the urine (*proteinuria*). It occurs in the second half of pregnancy, especially among first-time mothers, and can develop quite quickly. Sudden weight gain, perhaps caused by a sudden increase in water retention, can be a warning sign. Whilst toxemia tends to occur more commonly in overweight women, there is no evidence that excess weight gain in pregnancy is the actual cause. At one time, doctors would recommend a weight-reducing diet late in pregnancy if a mother had gained more than thirty pounds. In the early 1970s, however, it was clearly shown that this practice was both ineffective and dangerous. The best evidence came from Scottish researchers Campbell and MacGillivray, who showed that dieting did not alter the incidence of toxemia among first-time mothers who had gained excessive weight, but that it did cause a significant reduction in birth weight.[4] The babies had been virtually starved during the last weeks of pregnancy. A follow-up 4–6 years later showed that these babies had also continued to grow poorly. This was consistent with the findings of the United States National Institutes of Health, which had already shown that women who gained over 36 pounds had babies with the lowest level of brain damage or motor abnormalities.[2] The use of diuretics during pregnancy, which was once recommended to flush excessive water from the body, has similarly dropped out of fashion.[5]

If your sense of hunger seems to be functioning well and you seem to be getting a balanced diet, the chances are that you can safely trust yourself to eat the quantities you need. You probably eat whenever you are hungry and stop as soon as you feel you have had enough. If, however, you started the pregnancy obese, or severely underweight and perhaps anorexic, you will probably need to adjust your eating patterns.

PREGNANCY

Approximate average weight gain

lbs. and oz.

BABY:	10 weeks		20 weeks		30 weeks		40 weeks	
Fetus	0	¼	0	11	3	5	7	8
Placenta	0	¾	0	6	1	0	1	8
Amniotic fluid	0	1	0	3	1	10	1	10

MOTHER:								
Uterus	0	5	0	11	1	8	2	2
Breasts	0	1½	0	6	0	13	0	15
Blood	0	3½	1	5	1	13	2	9
Other fluids	0	0	0	1	0	3	3	10
Fat/protein stores	0	11	4	8	7	10	7	6
TOTALS: All tissue	1lb. 7oz.		8lb. 13oz.		17lb. 14oz.		27lb. 4oz.	

grams

BABY:	10 weeks	20 weeks	30 weeks	40 weeks
Fetus	5	300	1500	3400
Placenta	20	170	430	650
Amniotic fluid	30	350	750	800

MOTHER:				
Uterus	140	320	600	970
Breasts	45	180	360	405
Blood	100	600	1300	1250
Other fluids	0	30	80	1680
Fat/protein stores	310	2050	3480	3345
TOTALS: All tissue	650	4000	8500	12500

Overweight and underweight

Obesity is not a clearly defined condition. Broadly speaking, it means being grossly overweight with excessive fat layers round your body, and a weight-for-frame that is more than 120 percent of the Metropolitan Life ideal. The Metropolitan Life Insurance Company's 'ideal' weights are associated with the best chances of long life. If your pre-pregnancy weight was more than twenty percent above your ideal weight-for-frame size, as shown on the chart, you may have an overweight problem: and if you have rolls of fat around your hips and thighs and perhaps upper arms, you are almost certainly obese. If your pre-pregnancy weight was more than twenty percent below your weight-for-frame ideal, you may well be too light for good health.

Ideal weights for women (in pounds)
(Metropolitan Life Insurance Company)

Height Feet	Inches	Small Frame	Medium Frame	Large Frame
4	10	102–111	109–121	118–131
4	11	103–113	111–123	120–134
5	0	104–115	113–126	122–137
5	1	106–118	115–129	125–140
5	2	108–121	118–132	128–143
5	3	111–124	121–135	131–147
5	4	114–127	124–138	134–151
5	5	117–130	127–141	137–155
5	6	120–133	130–144	140–159
5	7	123–136	133–147	143–163
5	8	126–139	136–150	146–167
5	9	129–142	139–153	149–170
5	10	132–145	142–156	152–173
5	11	135–148	145–159	155–176
6	0	138–151	148–162	158–179

These ideal weights are for the age group 25–59; and they include indoor clothing and low-heeled shoes.[6]

Apart from the psychological difficulties that it tends to bring, obesity is associated with a number of physical disorders. In pregnancy, obesity means you are more likely to develop diabetes or toxemia, even though neither of these conditions has been shown to be *caused* by overeating. If you develop diabetes, you will almost certainly be put on a special diet, perhaps restricted in calories and with carefully controlled carbohydrate and fat intakes. If you do not have diabetes, but you either started pregnancy obese or seem to have becomer obese during it, a balanced diet now is very important.

Pregnancy is not the time for drastic weight-reducing diets, however. Such sudden stress could harm the fetus, as we have seen, and crash

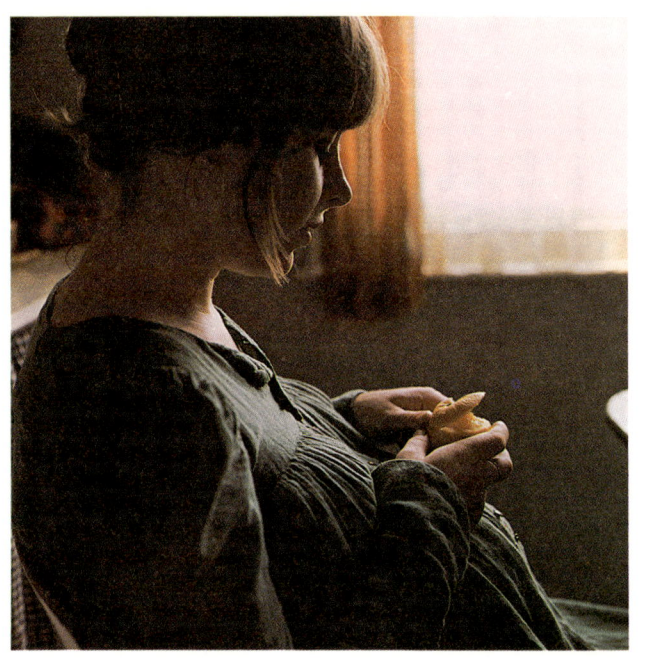

*Is your diet a healthy one?
Or is it time to change?*

dieting is anyway an ineffective way to lose weight on a long-lasting basis. But you *can* adjust to a balanced diet (as in the guidelines) by including relatively more whole grains, fresh vegetables and fruit, low-fat cheese and skimmed milk, while easing up on high-calorie fat-rich foods. This, together with plenty of walking, swimming, stretching, or simply weeding the garden should help you avoid any run-away weight-gain during the pregnancy.

Severe underweight is the converse of obesity. If you are eighty percent or less of the Metropolitan ideal for your height, then the chances are that you need to put on more than average weight during pregnancy. If you do not eat enough, your baby could be smaller than he might have been but, just as crash dieting is no good for pregnancy, forced eating is no solution either. You need to find a balance and this means being as truthful with yourself as you can be. Only if you can honestly say that you feel well at your present weight, and that you *do* eat as much as you want, is it sensible to trust your eating habits to provide what you and the baby need. If you sense that you are keeping your weight down because you are afraid of getting fat, or for any other reason, you may, without realizing it, be anorexic and you may need specialized medical help. Try the reverse of the guidelines for obese women. Eat more high-calorie, fat-rich foods like nuts, legumes, butter spreads, cheese, and cream. There is no sense in forcing it down, but do give yourself the chance to enjoy it.

Extreme overweight or extreme underweight can be so deeply ingrained in one's constitution that it becomes unalterable. The overweight tend to be slow burners of energy, often needing only normal amounts of food to maintain their high weight. They also usually take little exercise, which helps to keep them fat. In contrast, the constitutionally thin tend to be fast burners, often able to consume large quantities without putting on weight, their high activity level helping to keep them thin. But there are others whose abnormal weight is maintained only by distortions of hunger and appetite, so that they eat compulsively or regulate their food intake only by rigid self-control. Frequently these unnatural eating habits are of psychological origin.

Emotional eating disorders

Hilda Bruch, Professor of Psychiatry at Texas University, has been a pioneer in the understanding of emotional eating disorders. She defines those caught in such disorders as "individuals who misuse the eating function in their efforts to solve or camouflage problems of living"[7] and she makes it clear that of these problems, the emotional ones come high on the list: feelings of boredom or frustration, pent-up anger that never finds expression, loneliness, fear of the dark, fear of growing up, fear even of pleasure. Often these feelings have been encountered early in life and – because there was no apparent way to resolve them – they have been repressed, pushed back into the mind and the body. But they do not disappear. Rather, these unresolved emotions become masked by the less-specific, hard-to-identify but only just-below-the surface fear that we usually call *anxiety*.

Anxiety drives the human race to many bizarre, sometimes wonderful but far more often self-destructive activities. Overeating is one of the most common. Smoking, drinking, nail-biting, and anorexia (or combinations of them) are among the others. And what makes a person turn to eating in the face of anxiety is habit, often established in the very early years of life.

From your earliest days, your mother, or perhaps another nurturing adult, will have been your feeding partner, attending to your needs as best she could. If she understood you well, and was able to distinguish your cries of hunger from your other cries – of loneliness or anger, for example – you will have come to learn that *that* feeling (hunger) was appropriately satisfied by eating. As Hilda Bruch writes, "If things go well, a child will learn to identify his body needs correctly and to satisfy them in ways that are biologically appropriate". In this case, no disorder arises. If, however, you were trained to eat by the clock or to follow your mother's whims, your body's understanding may have been confused.

In early childhood, another set of influences is brought to bear on eating habits. The child in pain is often given sweets 'to make it better' or offered other snacks when bored or angry and starting to make more fuss than his parents care to stand. Most adults at some time or other are tempted to use food to keep a child quiet: and if this happens again and again, a child's true sense of hunger and appetite can become thoroughly confused. He eats whenever boredom or anger, loneliness, or pain occur. In this way, eating becomes a way of avoiding all kinds of uncomfortable feelings in an effort (albeit usually an unconscious one) to solve or camouflage the problems of life.

In adolescence, yet other influences may appear. Puberty may drive one girl out of overeating and another into it, for attitudes about menstruation and sexual encounters vary enormously. One girl is frightened and eats to cover herself with a protective layer of fat; another sheds her fat like an overcoat, hell-bent on slimming to model size. Yet another takes flight from sexual feelings by losing her appetite, which can delay menstruation. Nor are such changes usually conscious ones: they simply happen. However, through psychotherapy, family therapy, or even quiet reflection, the unconscious story can emerge.[8]

If you are caught up in emotional eating disorders, try to come to terms with them now, both for yourself and for your baby. Professional guidance may be necessary. Not only can unbalanced eating upset your developing baby now, it can also make feeding him in infancy more complicated: for a mother's habits are quickly passed on to her child.

Changing

By taking a closer look at your diet, you may well see your whole way of life more clearly, for the way we eat reflects the way we live. If you have decided that what you eat suits you well, and is providing well for the baby, you will feel little need to change. But if you have decided that certain changes are called for, more than your eating patterns will be involved. A break with old habits is always something of a personal revolution.

The best time to balance your diet is *before* you conceive. Your mate may well protest at first if you serve him salads or lightly cooked vegetables or wholewheat toast, if these are not his usual fare; but he may also take the opportunity to join you. If your diet seems to need changing and you can work at this together, there will be less chance of food conflict later on, when your baby starts to join you for meals at the family table.

Diet and pregnancy problems

Pregnancy calls for profound adaptation of the mother to the presence of the baby growing inside her. We have seen how the heart enlarges, the blood volume increases, digestion slows down, and the appetite becomes more sensitive, all apparently to enhance the harmonious growth of the baby. These adaptations are associated with equally radical changes in metabolism. In the process of these changes, many women experience nausea, heartburn, and raised blood pressure, and a few develop toxemia. Such problems are all, to some degree, associated with what you eat.

Morning sickness

Morning sickness, as millions of mothers know, can go on all day, every day, for weeks and even months on end. Some pregnant women feel queasy on rising but return to normal during the morning. Many others experience a more-or-less constant state of nausea. In most cases, the condition starts during early pregnancy and disappears by the fourth month: sometimes, however, it continues until the birth.

Every science concerned with pregnancy has suggested possible causes of this ancient and common phenomenon. Genetic inheritance, lifestyle and diet before conception, anxiety, frequent unwanted sexual intercourse, and the mother's unconscious attitude towards the baby have all been implicated. As it occurs primarily in the first three months of pregnancy and because it is so common – approximately half of all pregnant women suffer from it[1] – morning sickness is probably part of the mother's natural adaptation to her fetus. It certainly forces many women who might otherwise be rushing about as usual to slow down. This may even be why the rate of spontaneous abortions is lower among women who do have some nausea.[2,3]

There are no well-established cures for morning sickness other than those the body demands for itself: rest, sleep, and very little food. You are likely to know exactly what you can stomach in the way of food, which is commonly regular small snacks. Fatty foods are usually unacceptable.

Vitamin B_6 has gained the reputation of relieving pregnancy nausea and may be effective for women who are already mildly deficient in B_6 at conception, especially if they have been taking the contraceptive pill which increases requirements for this vitamin.[4] Up to 50 milligrams daily (starting with 10 milligrams and gradually increasing the dose over a week or so) may help. Good food sources of B_6 include wholewheat bread, brown rice, liver, nuts, herrings, salmon and, if you can stomach it, blackstrap molasses.

Among herbal remedies long used for pregnancy nausea are spearmint, lobelia, and the red raspberry leaf. According to the 19th century Wisconsin-born natural healer Jethro Kloss, red raspberry leaves made into tea is good to relieve nausea and vomiting, and is an effective aid to uterine contractions in labor.[5]

If you experience severe nausea during pregnancy, the only thing you will probably feel like doing is relaxing. The rest of the household will have to make fewer demands on you, especially as you may not feel like cooking for them, or even eating with them. Indeed, you may want to be looked after yourself. You will also probably find it necessary to lie down – preferably in the fresh air – for at least part of the day. To ease the discomfort when you do so, practice breathing fairly deeply (but always gently).

If you start vomiting, it may be best to consult your doctor. Prolonged vomiting can be a serious condition as there is a risk of excess water and nutrient loss. But it is also worth remembering that the symptoms of nausea are known sometimes to have emotional causes.[6]

Heartburn

Heartburn is a form of indigestion caused by regurgitation of part of the stomach contents up towards the throat. The acid fluid that rises – in pregnancy, often as a result of uterine pressure on the stomach – causes a burning sensation in the region of the heart. In the short term, antacids can be helpful, and their occasional use appears to be quite safe,[6,7] but long term use is not without hazards: sodium bicarbonate may cause salt overloading, calcium carbonate can lead to excessively high calcium levels in the blood and to kidney damage, and aluminium hydroxide may result in phosphate depletion.[8] In his review of the available drugs, Professor Murray Enkin of the McMaster University Medical School in Ontario, considers magnesium salts the safest.[7] In the longer term, you may need to eat smaller, more frequent meals that do not fill your stomach. Lemon verbena and camomile infusions, available as tea bags, may be helpful. They are a delicious substitute for tea and coffee.

High blood pressure

High blood pressure, especially during the early months of pregnancy, is a warning sign. Moderate hypertension carries no risk, except insofar as it may become more severe and lead to toxemia.[9] A diet too rich in salt or protein, and perhaps in saturated fatty acid foods like meat fat, cream, and butter, is known to contribute to high blood pressure in some women. And so is stress.

If your blood pressure has been creeping up or suddenly rises, you will need to watch your diet.

Follow the guidelines, making sure that you avoid very salty foods, especially cured meats, smoked fish, and highly salted butter or cheese, which tend to provide too much salt and saturated fats. You need not become a vegetarian, but remember that vegetarians tend *not* to develop high blood pressure, and this is in part due to their diet.[10] Nor should you cut salt out of your diet completely. In fact, this could make matters worse. Extreme salt restriction can damage your kidneys and has been associated in one study with an *increased* rate of toxemia.[11] You can also improve your ability to cope with stress – and your general health – by taking up yoga, stretching, or some other form of active relaxation.

Toxemia

Pregnant women suffering from nausea, hypertension, water retention (*edema*) and a high urinary excretion of protein (*proteinuria*) are said to have *toxemia* or *pre-eclampsia*. Mild toxemia carries no immediate risk, but it can, if not treated, lead to *eclampsia*, a major threat to both mother and baby. Regular pre-natal checkups are the best way to ensure that you are not affected by such symptoms as these

There is no one known cause of the various symptoms of toxemia. A number of metabolic disorders, kidney disease, a parasitic worm, and an unbalanced diet have all been implicated, but none of them is firmly established as the cause. For many years, it was commonly believed that toxemia could be controlled by severely restricting salt intake (salt was thought to be the cause of the water retention); but this is now known to be quite ineffective and even harmful.[11] However, do try not to eat too many highly salted foods like cheese and pickles, cured meats, and smoked fish. Weight control by strict dieting and the use of diuretics to reduce the edema were also both once commonly recommended but are now discredited: both are, in fact, ineffective and potentially harmful.[11,12]

Other aspects of diet have also been implicated: too little protein, for example: and a high-protein diet has been recommended for toxemia. However, Professor David Rush of the Albert Einstein College of Medicine in New York has reported that poorly nourished mothers have lighter babies if they get a protein-rich supplement, but heavier babies if the supplements contain a more balanced range of nutrients.[13] So there does appear to be some risk in suddenly stuffing yourself with protein, and very little evidence that eating more protein reduces the chances that you will develop toxemia.

Vitamin and mineral supplements have also long been recommended for toxemia, although the evidence supporting this practice is sparse. One well-publicized study in London in 1942 showed that women given supplements had a lower incidence of toxemia.[14,15] However, the mortality rate of the babies of these same supplemented mothers was higher than for the babies of women who received no supplements. It is not easy to interpret this sort of information. More recently, claims have been made that Vitamin B_6 and folic acid are helpful in preventing toxemia.

Whatever the causes of toxemia, it is clear that the place of diet is controversial. At present we cannot with any confidence recommend anything but a well-balanced diet during pregnancy, together with low-level supplementation for those who may have become deficient before they conceived. This includes a good supply of all vitamins and minerals, and a moderate salt intake.

Provided that blood pressure does not continue to rise, toxemia is normally nothing worse than a warning. Rest is generally considered essential, and hospital admission is frequently recommended. Over the last thirty years, a number of drugs have been used to control blood pressure, among the latest being *methyldopa* and, in some instances, the *beta blockers* prescribed for non-pregnancy hypertension, but their use is still controversial.

If your blood pressure is increasing, or your legs begin to swell, or you feel sick, you should be resting periodically throughout the day. Your doctor will certainly advise this. Eat plenty of whole grains and vegetables (cooked or raw). Cut processed refined foods completely out of your diet for a while; and switch from tea, coffee, colas and alcohol to herbal teas and bottled water. Spring water, bottled at source, sometimes called mineral water, is free of the residues of antibacterial chemicals. Though not essential, it probably adds to the therapeutic value of the diet. And it usually tastes better than tap water.

Eclampsia

If toxemia continues without being treated, there is a risk of *eclampsia* developing. Any nausea experienced may grow into migraine, with symptoms of visual disturbance and headache. Water retention may spread to the face, vulva, arms, and hands, and the blood pressure may increase further. There may finally be epileptic-like fits and coma. Thanks to improved pre-natal care, eclampsia is now relatively rare, but it is still a major risk to both mother and baby when it does occur. If blood pressure can be controlled, and there are no signs of fetal distress, delivery is postponed on a day-to-day basis in the hospital: but because of the high risks, induction of labor or caesarian section is the normal outcome.[9]

To breast or bottle-feed?

During the last months of the pregnancy, you are likely to be thinking more and more of the birth and, if this is your first baby, of how you are going to handle the first few weeks after it. One of the decisions you will soon have to make is how you will feed your baby. Because your choice will profoundly affect his future and the future of your relationship with him, this is a question to be considered *now*, while you still have time to reflect at leisure. Today, most mothers probably know that breastfeeding is best and the number who give it a try has increased enormously over the last ten years: yet most milk fed to young babies in our society still comes from a factory.[1]

The reasons for this are largely historical. Bottle-feeding is, after all, a child of the technological age, an age that reached a particular peak during the 1950s and 1960s. In this age of scientific optimism, the formula seemed to be an utterly reliable, sensible, hygienic, and convenient way to feed one's baby. The medical profession endorsed it. Breastfeeding came to be seen as something vulgar, perhaps even bestial, fine for animals but not for *us*! Urged on by a growing infant-food industry, and encouraged in the hospital to bottle-feed after the birth, the vast majority of mothers twenty years ago did not even try to breastfeed. But the tide turned. A massive body of evidence gradually built up to show the potential risks associated with formula-feeding and the previously unknown benefits of breastfeeding. By 1975, a movement back to breastfeeding was under way.

Breast milk

Breast milk is a living fluid made from the mother's own blood, that same blood that fed the baby in the womb. So it clearly offers a natural continuation of exactly that kind of nourishment that your baby was used to in the womb. Like the blood, breast milk continually varies in composition, not only in response to the mother's lifestyle and diet, but also in response to the changing needs of the growing baby. It varies from day to day, from feed to feed and from one part of the feed to another, as part of the complex, constantly changing exchange between mother and child. No two women follow exactly the same pattern: each has her own unique milk.[2] But it has been established that the milk of a well-nourished mother can provide the baby's entire diet during his first year of life.[3]

Breast milk also protects the baby from a broad range of illnesses. The milk contains antibodies to disease, proteins taken from the mother's blood, called *immunoglobulins*. Very high concentrations pass from mother to baby just before the birth (in the blood) and just afterwards (in the first milk, known as *colostrum*).[4]

Another form of protection, and nourishment, that comes with breastfeeding is an emotional or psychological one. For breastfeeding is the scene of the most personal exchanges between mother and baby and provides the foundation of their relationship. Scientists have called this relationship the *mother-baby bond* and sometimes speak of *bonding* as the process whereby each comes to meet the other after the birth. Breastfeeding is a tremendously important part of the bonding process. Well-bonded babies appear to develop greater emotional stability and intellectual ability as they grow older than those babies who lack the stimulation of a close physical and emotional relationship with their mothers which is enhanced by breastfeeding.[5,6]

From the mother's point-of-view, breastfeeding has yet other advantages. For a start, it is far easier than bottle-feeding: there are no bottles, nipples, jugs, spoons and sterilizing equipment to cope with. It is safer than bottle-feeding, too, because the milk passes straight from the breast into the baby's mouth without exposure to germs in the air. And breastfeeding is, of course, cheaper: in fact, it is free – yet another practical advantage in times of economic difficulties.

If you think you would like to breastfeed but feel anxious about it – perhaps afraid you will not have enough milk, or that it will hurt you or spoil your figure – use the rest of your pregnancy to come to terms with your feelings and to find out all you can about it.

Bottled milk

Although breast is best, many women still prefer to bottle-feed. Like most nutritionists, we would recommend you not to bottle-feed, but it is only fair to say that millions of healthy children have been fed this way, and for many of them the experience seems to have been satisfactory. There are, however, certain risks attached to formula-feeding, as we shall see, and this is particularly so in the poorest countries.

Bottled milk or formula – so named because it is made according to a precise chemical formula – is a synthetic substitute for breast milk. Usually based on cows' milk, but containing many additional chemical ingredients, the latest formulas contain more-or-less the same proportions of protein, fat, carbohydrate, minerals, and vitamins as breast milk. But the taste, the texture, and the effect on the baby are rather different. And unlike the mother's milk, which varies in composition depending on the baby's changing requirements, bottled milk is always the same in its consistency and content, providing it is correctly mixed.

As for the risks, bottle-fed babies have more feeding problems, more infections, and more allergies.[7,8] And in very poor Third World countries, where drinking water is often contaminated, bottle-feeding can be fatal.[9] In addition, formula-fed babies tend to grow faster and fatter than breastfed babies,[10,11] while bottle-feeding mothers (who do not use their breasts for nursing) appear to be more at risk for breast cancer later in life,[12] though how much more at risk is not yet known.

The first scientifically designed formula came from the laboratories of the German, J. von Liebig in 1867. An elderly theoretical chemist, he was only known to conduct one study of living subjects in his whole life, so his formula was far removed from reality. It was made from milk, wheat flour, malt flour and sodium bicarbonate, a mixture that could not be legally marketed today as a baby milk.

By the 1950s, dried cows' milk, with added iron and Vitamins A and D, was in common use as infant formula. Doctors endorsed it. Yet by the early 1970s, it was clear that the high mineral content strained some babies' kidneys;[13] that the butterfat of cows' milk was very poorly absorbed, causing diarrhea and weight loss in some babies; and that the protein content was too high, causing excessive weight gain.[14] It had become obvious that a new sort of formula was required.

On medical advice, the manufacturers changed their products, and by the later 1970s a new range of so-called *humanized milks* (even more like breast milk) was on the market. Vegetable oils were used instead of the butterfat; the protein concentration was reduced; and the whey itself was electrochemically demineralized to reduce the excess mineral salt levels, before being refortified with selected minerals, such as zinc, copper and magnesium, at the levels in which they occur in breast milk.

These new products are the best that can be manufactured given the current limitations in scientific knowledge and production technology. But they pose a number of important questions concerning safety in use. One manufacturer has commented: "Except possibly for the case of iron, neither the physiological response of the young infant nor the toxicology of the mineral salts is well known".[15]

Doubts have also been raised about the vegetable oils in the humanized formulas. Although better absorbed than butterfat, they lack the cholesterol that is found in both cows' and human milk. In the 1970s, when cholesterol was strongly associated with heart disease, this lack of cholesterol from the formula was seen as an advantage. Critics have subsequently pointed out, however, that babies probably *need* the cholesterol in breast milk for healthy nerve tissue, and perhaps to induce the development of enzymes that break down dietary cholesterol in later life.[16,17] There is indeed some evidence that adults who were bottle-fed as babies seem to have higher cholesterol levels than those who were breastfed.[18] These adults also have abnormally high levels of antibodies to cows' milk proteins in their blood.[19] So it could be that bottle-feeding is yet another contributory cause of heart disease in later life, although this is not yet proven.

Yet for babies whose mothers are unable to breastfeed, the formulas are lifesaving. They are manufactured as carefully as any medical drugs and are as important to our health services. The trouble is that they have increasingly become the norm, like much of the medical technology developed over the last thirty years or so for the management of birth.

The birth connection

In most hospitals, birth has become a technological event, where the management of labor involves routine episiotomy (cutting the perineum), routine early clamping of the umbilical cord and separation of mother and baby after delivery, and extremely high rates of induction, anesthesia, and caesarian section. In most hospitals, free samples of formula are also given to new mothers, despite international codes to the contrary.[20] And in some hospitals, the personnel continue to insist on giving supplementary feedings of formula to breastfed babies. All these practices, during and after labor, carry some risk to either mother or child, or both. Yet they are frequently used as part of the routine, often for no other reason than convenience.[21,22] We share the increasingly common view that these practices should be used only for their true purpose, as a stand-by procedure to be used only if something goes wrong.[22]

There are millions of mothers who could, if given the encouragement and support, deliver and breastfeed their babies quite naturally, as our ancestors have done over millions of years. The knowledge that facilities are available if something goes wrong can only be reassuring. There are several organizations that provide support for women who want an 'active' or 'natural' birth, as well as groups offering instruction and guidance for breastfeeding, such as the La Leche League. If you think you would like to adopt this approach, make contact with a group that can help you. If you think you would like to breastfeed but have some reservations about it, give some time to reflecting on your deeper feelings about it. Sometimes bottle-feeding, with all its problems, can be avoided if only these feelings can be brought to light in time. For negative feelings can spoil any attempt to breastfeed.

Feelings about breastfeeding

The reasons why breastfeeding is best are clear enough: but it is *feelings* that decide whether breastfeeding can actually succeed. It takes more than the wagging finger of a well-meaning nurse to establish lactation! Many women start to breastfeed in the hospital, but the vast majority switch to the bottle within days of returning home. For many of these mothers, feelings of anxiety commonly disturb the self-confidence that is an all important requirement for successful breastfeeding.[1]

Some are afraid that breastfeeding will ruin their figures; others that their breasts will never be able to provide all the milk required. Some are ashamed of their breasts and want to keep them hidden away, even feeling disgusted by the very idea of a baby sucking at their nipples. Others fear that breastfeeding will cut them off from the rest of the world. If we lived in close communities as our ancestors did, and indeed many people throughout the world still do, we would be quite accustomed to the sight of mothers suckling their young. Nowadays, however, millions of mothers and fathers-to-be have grown up without ever having seen a baby being fed in what is the natural way. How much more familiar to see a bottle in a baby's mouth!

The way *you* were fed as a child and the nature of your sex education may hold some clues to discovering just why you may be experiencing anxiety and uncertainty about breastfeeding. It may help, therefore, to spend a while looking back to your own early years.

The mother as a child

The way in which a mother feeds her baby can affect their relationship in the most profound and lasting way. So deep are these first impressions that years later, when the baby herself becomes a mother-to-be, they may strongly color her own attitude towards feeding. If you were given all the breast milk you needed as a baby, you will probaby feel positive about breastfeeding your own children. If you were denied access to your mother's breast, however, and had to make do with a rubber nipple instead, you may well feel more distant from your mother, and perhaps intend to bottle-feed. The memories of early experience, including satisfaction at being close to your mother or the frustrations of not being close enough, remain in the unconscious mind.[2] In order to make the connection between how you were fed as a baby and how you feel about feeding your own baby, you may need to reflect a little. Concentrate on how you feel about your own mother's breasts and take note of these feelings: compare this with how you feel about your own breasts. Consider whether you had what you needed from your mother and how much you intend to give to your own child once he is born. There is likely to be a strong connection between what was done for you by your mother in your own early infancy and what you feel like doing for your baby.

Many a pregnant woman is drawn towards her own mother during the sometimes bewildering months before and after birth. Take advantage of the situation to find out what you can about *her* experience when you, and perhaps also your brothers and sisters, were born and *her* attitude towards breastfeeding. It may help you to understand something of the mothering you received from her so long ago.

You might also consider your reaction when your own breasts began to grow. Were you pleased and proud or did you try to hide them? How you felt at that time was probably a reflection of how you felt about becoming a woman. Was sex something talked about openly in your home or was it a taboo subject? For many, there is still an embarrassment, even shame, about the three great sexual events of life – making love, giving birth and breastfeeding. Your breasts, like the rest of you, are uniquely your own. No breast is too large or too small for feeding. If you lack confidence, you will certainly find it comforting to talk with the breastfeeding mothers you meet, or with someone from one of the breastfeeding organizations. Seek all the advice and guidance you can. It should help enormously to assuage any doubts.

Is breastfeeding inconvenient?

First-time pregnant women sometimes express the fear that the baby will utterly disrupt their lives, and hope to minimize this disruption by using a bottle 'that anyone can give'. You may have a job and want to get back to it as soon after the birth as possible; you may have other commitments; or you may be worried that breastfeeding will set you apart socially. While it is quite likely that motherhood *will* radically change your life, it does not necessarily follow that breastfeeding will isolate you or stop you from working, nor that bottle-feeding would make everyday life any easier at all in the months prior to weaning your baby.

In some countries, women are given paid maternity leave from work, but usually they are left to make their own arrangements. For the many single women who have children there is often no choice: they *have* to work. If you would like to breastfeed but cannot avoid returning to work, try to arrange that the baby is not too far away, so that you can go to him at feeding time. Some dedicated mothers manage another approach, expressing their milk and leaving it to be fed to the baby in a bottle while they are absent. This enables them to be away for a good part of the day: and because expressing milk, like sucking, has the effect of stimulating lactation, it helps to keep the milk supply strong for breastfeeding for those times when the mother *is* at home with her baby.

Breastfeeding can be done virtually anywhere with a minimum of fuss. You can very quickly learn to find a quiet spot and to feed so that not even an inch of your breast is visible to the rest of the world, if this is worrying to you.

Breast shape and feeding

Most women find that after prolonged breastfeeding – by this we mean a year or more for each child – their breasts are slightly smaller and less firm than in the days before motherhood. Some are disappointed with this change, but many others welcome it.

The process begins soon after conception. In fact, a tight, full feeling in the breasts is one of the earliest signs of pregnancy. If you previously had very small breasts, this could be an extra bonus to the pregnancy: if you have always been on the heavy side, it could be uncomfortable. By the time of the birth, most women's breasts are as large as they have ever been. This is the body's natural preparation for breastfeeding.

After the birth, once feeding is under way, the breasts are regularly filled with milk and emptied by the baby. This rhythmic stretching and shrinking of the tissue gradually reduces its former firmness to some extent, but this can be minimized by exercise and good posture. If you are used to wearing a bra, you can obtain special breastfeeding models that open at the front. If you do not normally wear a bra, you may well have realized that the shape of your breasts depends very much on the way you stand and sit: an erect spine and open shoulders raise the breast-line, while a slumped spine and closed shoulders lower it. One way to release the tension in tight, closed shoulders is to stretch them every day. Properly supervised stretching or hatha yoga provides a wonderful preparation for birth itself, acting as an antidote for the stresses of family life and improving both your figure and your posture.[3,4]

The father's point of view

Your baby's father, sharing the pregnancy with you, can also play an important part in your choice of how to feed the baby. What he says about breastfeeding and, more important, what he *feels* about it, may make a great difference. For he is not simply a bystander: he was also once a baby, calling for his mother's breast, and he unconsciously remembers all about it. If he was breastfed, he may encourage you to do the same for his child; if he was not, he may try to dissuade you. There are also those, of course, who were not breastfed themselves but who very much want their own children to have a different experience of early feeding.

The ease with which you talk about feeding will depend on the nature of your relationship, and so will your final choice. If you find yourselves in disagreement, try to get to the root of it now, or there may be feeding problems later on when the baby senses the conflict, as he probably will.

Men sometimes find it extremely difficult to express their feelings, or even to know exactly what they do feel. Emotional freedom is not a part of most men's education. On the contrary, boys are often expected to bottle up their feelings, especially the tender ones, which are commonly considered effeminate. Men are expected to be rational, firmly based in the world of reason rather than in the world of emotions. So you may have to use all your tact and good humor to draw him into an honest conversation about the whole subject of whether or not you will breastfeed your baby and for how long. This may be something you can achieve quickly or it may take weeks.

At first, your discussions may be very reasonable, 'reasons' being a man's more familiar mental territory. If he does not feel good about breastfeeding, he may say that it will ruin your figure, or that it is not 'nice' or that it is not necessary. Try to lead him into talking about his feelings. How does he feel about the prospect of the baby sucking at your breasts? Perhaps he has the unconscious feeling that your breasts 'belong' to him, even that *you* belong to him! Many fathers-to-be are jealous of the unborn baby without consciously realizing it. If you suspect this is the case, try to find out how he feels about the baby in other respects. Encourage him to feel the fetal movements and to talk to the baby, even at a fairly early stage in your pregnancy. If he is jealous, perhaps you can help to reassure him with affection so that it becomes apparent that this is neither a helpful nor a reasonable reaction.

A first pregnancy is often a major test of the parents' relationship. For as the months pass, it becomes increasingly obvious that you are no longer two, but three. Take advantage of the months that remain to adapt to the fact. The father who gets involved with his child before the birth, and prepares for it with you, will more easily find his place with you during labor, making the event a happier, easier one for you all. And if he sees the birth, the chances are he will be that much more sensitive to the newborn baby, which may well make him a good ally in breastfeeding.

Preparations for feeding

Look after your body: it is the temple of your spirit. Examine it in a mirror and with your hands. Admire your better parts, but give even more attention to those you like less. If you take care of them, you may find they brighten up. After a bath, enjoy the luxury of rubbing your whole body slowly with a cream or oil. If you intend to breastfeed, give special attention to your breasts. Massage them with a little almond or wheatgerm oil every few days, gently but firmly kneading them between thumb and forefinger. Then stroke them towards the nipple. Later on in the pregnancy, you may even find a drop of milky fluid emerges. There is no need to bathe your breasts with alcohol during pregnancy, as some draconian authorities insisted in the past, nor to scrub them with a brush. Even the use of soap is not recommended, as it removes the natural oils produced by the skin. Caring for your breasts now should help prevent them from becoming engorged or inflamed during early feeding.

Inverted nipples may make breastfeeding more difficult, but there are things you can do to make them more prominent. Partly inverted nipples sometimes start to project quite spontaneously towards the end of pregnancy, but you can help the process along with gentle massage or during love-making. If your nipples are completely inverted, you may need to wear special plastic shields during the second half of the pregnancy. They are sometimes effective in pressing the nipples forward. Start by wearing them for just an hour each day, and gradually work up during pregnancy to about six hours.

There is in fact not a muscle or joint in your body that would not benefit from tender, firm massage. Make sure you get plenty of rest, too: you will need to be fit for the birth, and the inevitable broken nights that come after it. If you work, try to spend five minutes, every hour or two, relaxing. There are many ways to do this.

One simple method is to sit down, close your eyes, and turn your thoughts inwards. At least once a day, too, try to find a quiet place and lie down on the floor with a couple of pillows, end-to-end, underneath your spine. If you should feel at all dizzy, turn on your side.

If you want to breastfeed and your baby is to be born in hospital, make sure that your file there contains notes about your intention. Many hospitals routinely give newborn babies supplementary feedings of formula, so the note in your file should read 'Wants to breastfeed

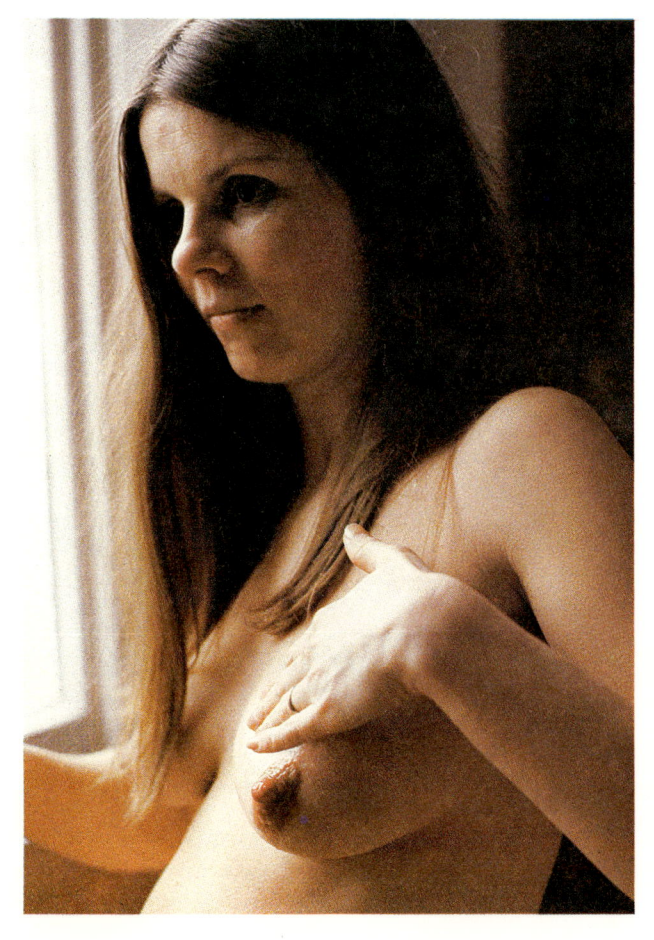

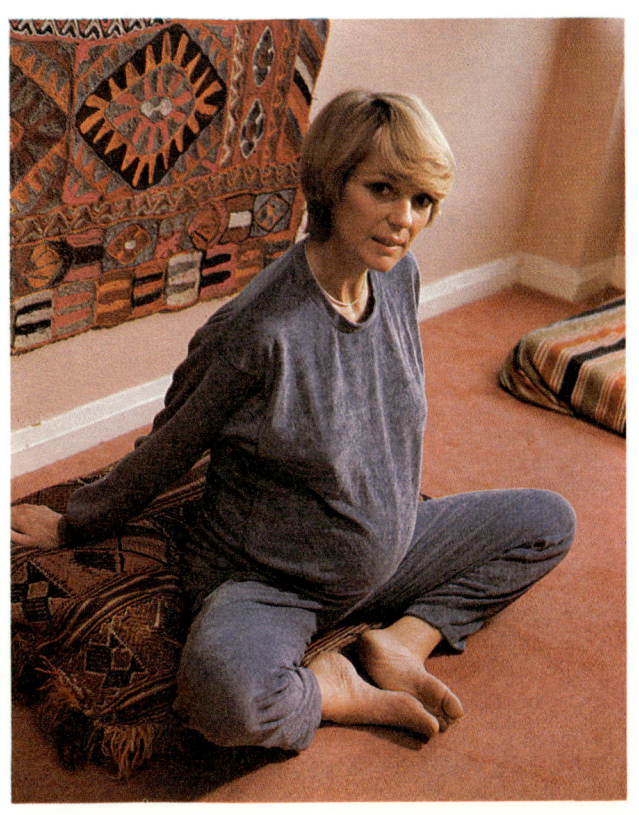

Breast care will aid feeding, and a pre-natal exercise program will prepare you for the birth.

Preparations for feeding

entirely'. Your wishes about the way you would prefer to give birth should be entered in the same file. And when you get to the hospital, make sure the nurses or staff know what has been arranged. It may even be helpful to have a card with you, reading 'Breastfeeding only. Mother available any time, day or night'. This can be stuck to the baby's crib.

Illness need not prevent you from breastfeeding, although some ongoing conditions – such as heart or kidney disease, cancer, tuberculosis or diabetes – may make bottle-feeding preferable. Your doctor may be able to advise on this. Short-term illnesses like influenza or mild infections need not stand in your way, though they may reduce the amount of milk you produce. Caesarian section can also make breastfeeding harder to get going, but certainly need not prevent it.

Preparations for bottle-feeding

If you feel more at ease with the idea of bottle-feeding, then this is probably the best path for you to take. Your baby is likely to be better off if you are relaxed and bottle-feeding than if you are tense and breastfeeding.

Everything recommended as a preparation for breastfeeding will also help those who intend to use a bottle. Looking after yourself now will serve to make the pregnancy and the birth easier, while the potentially trying months of your early relationship with your baby will be more fun and less of a burden if you are fit.

The most common problems associated with bottle-feeding (digestive disturbances, allergic reactions, and infections) will probably keep you in closer contact with your doctor or health visitor than would otherwise have been the case. But you can minimize the risk of these and other problems by paying careful attention to hygiene when making up the feedings, and by holding your baby close when feeding because bottle-fed babies tend to lack that important early physical contact.

If you do decide to bottle-feed, try to give breast milk for the first week or two if you can, and then gradually phase it out over a period of several days. This way, your baby will benefit from the immunity to disease provided by certain proteins in your milk. And if you think you will need to leave the baby with someone else for a large part of the day, take the time now to find someone who is really fond of babies and who will give a bottle to your infant, as you would, with much love.

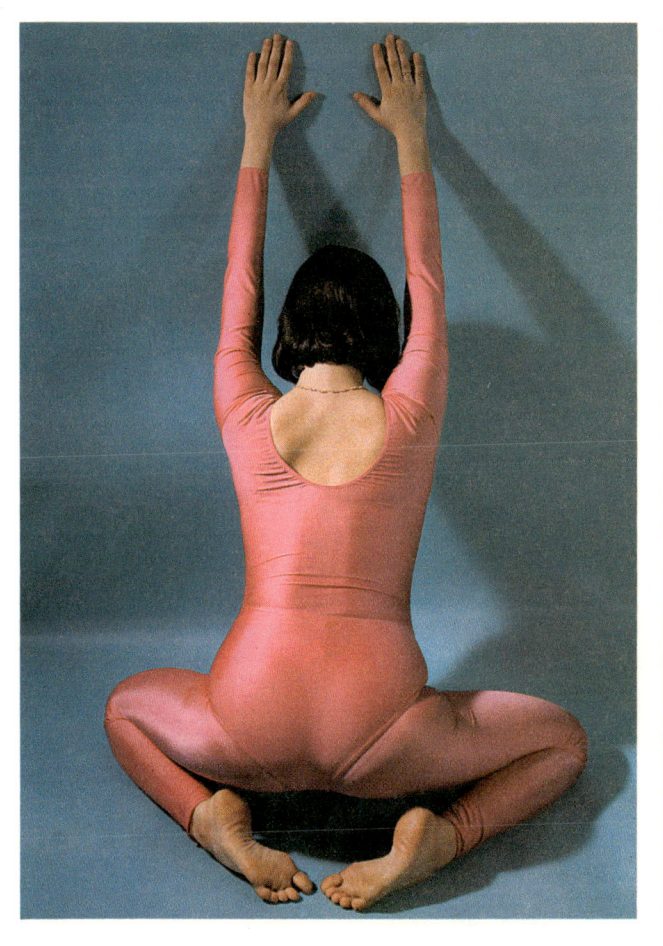

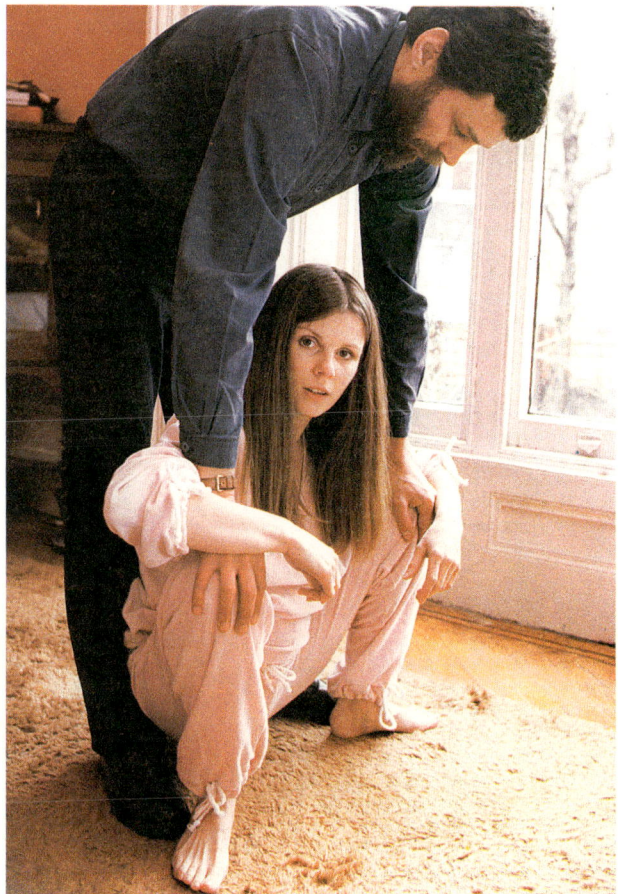

The birth

The pregnancy draws to term and, cramped within the womb, the mature fetus waits, fully prepared for his journey to the outer world. Food and oxygen still pump along the umbilical vein, but his digestive and respiratory systems are ready now to function independently. His kidneys are still not quite mature, nor is his brain: but he can see, hear, taste, and feel with the utmost sensitivity.[1]

Just as your baby is physically ready to be born, so you are probably ready to deliver him. For nine months your body has carried and fed him: and for many weeks, you have been preparing for the birth, talking with doctors, nurses, midwives, other mothers and friends, learning breathing techniques for labor, preparing the nursery. Now you probably want to get on with it.

Childbirth is potentially the most exciting event in your life, a confirmation of your deepest female nature. The more positive you feel, the more likely it is that all will go well.

Do everything you can to make it as happy an event as possible. Approach it in a spirit of hope. It was Sheila Kitzinger, the British anthropologist and childbirth teacher, who inspired many of our generation to regard childbirth in this way. "Pain in labor", she writes, "is real enough. We dare not underestimate the agony that some unprepared women endure in childbirth . . . But when a woman has her baby happily, she spreads a different spirit – a mood of gladness rather than the dread and horror that is associated with most old wives' tales . . . It is this spirit of hope, this joy of birth as a fulfilment of a man and woman's love for each other that should be the essence of birth."[2]

The natural event

Consider the natural event of birth. Your uterus, a massive muscle, begins to ripple, contracting and expanding, gently at first, then more and more energetically. Prepared, you will know how to face the discomfort and how to enjoy the rests, breathing and riding the storm. Inside the womb, your baby will also be having an awesome experience as the warm waters drain away and he is pressed with a magnificent rhythmical force along the birth canal.

And then, after what may be many hours, he emerges into the dry, cooler air of the outside world. Though still receiving oxygen through the umbilical cord, his lungs begin to breathe. He gives a cry of wonder, excitement and alarm, but almost immediately his slippery skin feels yours, and the warmth and softness of your body reassure him. After some minutes, the silvery cord stops pulsing and is clamped, then cut. Perhaps you lift your baby onto your breasts, at last face to face with him. He may begin to suck, which releases hormones in your body that make the uterus contract again, helping to expel the placenta, and stimulating the production in your breasts of your first milk.

This ancient process is sometimes called *natural birth* or, when the mother is free to move about as she pleases and to deliver the child in any position that suits her, *active birth*. This sort of birth is a very personal event, with its own particular timing.

Hospital management

There has been much debate about the hospital management of labor. Do the benefits of modern obstetrics outweigh the hazards?[3] Hardly a step in the birth process escapes controversy. Do mothers *need* an enema? *Why* must the pubic hair be shaved? Is it proper to induce labor simply for the convenience of the hospital staff? Is it safe? Does routine *episiotomy* – the cutting of the perineum 'in case the mother tears' – cause more harm than good?[4] *Should* the umbilical cord be cut before it has stopped pulsing? Why should babies be separated from their mothers after delivery, when they ought to be together? And do women not have a right to know what facilities are available, in order to assess for themselves the pros and cons? These questions are being asked and discussed more and more commonly, and hospital routines are gradually changing as a result. For there is evidence that routine intervention in birth can itself be a cause of complications.[3]

Two French obstetricians, Frederick Leboyer and Michel Odent, in their respective maternity clinics near Paris, have shown that very sparing use of modern technology, together with a deep respect for the mother's intuitive wishes during labor, is not only courteous but clinically safer and the best way to help her have an easy labor. Their record of birth without complications is astonishingly good.[5]

These developments in obstetrics reach deeply into the field of nutrition. For the quality of the birth affects the quality of all that follows. For those mothers who enjoy an uncomplicated birth in the hospital, breastfeeding usually comes with ease: but for those who do not, breastfeeding can be hard to establish. Induction, anesthesia, and episiotomy, for example – all at one time used only when really necessary – have now become commonplace and even routine: and all may hamper breastfeeding. The American Academy of Pediatrics has recommended "a decrease in the amount of anesthesia and/or sedation given to the mother during labor and delivery because large amounts can impair the baby's sucking".[6]

The early clamping of the umbilical cord after

the delivery may also affect the nutrition of the baby, but in a rather different way. Under normal circumstances, the cord continues to carry oxygen and other nutrients to the newborn until his lungs have established their breathing. As it is some twenty inches long, the cord can do this even when the baby has been born and is some distance from the placenta. But hospital routine usually dictates that the cord be cut as soon as the baby is out. The nutritional effect of this is prematurely to cut off the baby's food supply. As long ago as 1892, it was known that the level of iron-containing hemoglobin in the blood of babies whose cords were not immediately clamped was considerably higher than that of the 'early–clamped' babies, and that their weight gain during the first week was better. In 1959, the British Medical Research Council reported that a full-term baby whose cord is clamped five minutes after birth receives about 50 grams more blood from the placenta than if the cord is cut after thirty seconds:[7] this amounts to about three months supply of iron and other minerals.

There is one more routine, still practiced in some hospitals, that tends to have detrimental effect on early feeding: the separation of mother and baby immediately after the birth.

Hospital routine commonly dictates that the baby is taken away after the delivery: to draw the mucus from his nose, to mark him with a bracelet, to weigh and measure him, to wash the protective vernix from his skin and to wrap him in a sterile towel. Only then are mother and baby allowed a token meeting before the infant is whisked off for a physical examination and a place in the nursery, separated from his mother so that she can 'get some rest'. Avoid this procedure if you can. There is now a good deal of evidence that a baby who is with his mother during the first hours after birth subsequently has a different sort of relationship with her. For something seems to pass between a mother and her child during their first face to face encounters after delivery, an exchange that unites the two in a deeply empathetic relationship and evokes in the mother a profound attachment for her child. The technical term for this process of attachment is *bonding*, and it is an important ingredient of breastfeeding. Bonding is not something that occurs *only* during the first hours after the birth, but its development does appear to go through a crucial stage at that time.

Sheep farmers have long known of this critical period after the birth. If a new born lamb is immediately taken from the ewe and returned thirty minutes later, the mother will butt and kick it away when the two are reunited. In contrast, if they are left together after the birth but separated two days later for an equal period of time, their relationship is unaffected. Human mothers may not butt their babies away when they meet them after a delay, but the mothering instinct may be dulled and breastfeeding may be harder to get going.

Ask to have your baby with you from the start. He can be washed and weighed later. Other than in an emergency, *nothing* is more important than for the two of you to be together.[8]

Overcoming obstacles

Most births in the West take place in the hospital and, if you are well prepared and the staff are sympathetic, the experience can be a good one. Despite the shortcomings of some of the routine procedures, many women prefer to know that, should anything go wrong, medical facilities are near at hand. If, however, you feel enough confidence to give birth at home and your doctor says there are no contraindications, and you can find all the assistance you need to do so, you may prefer to arrange for a home birth. In Holland, where the percentage of home births is the highest in the western world, the perinatal mortality rate is among the lowest.[9]

If you are having a hospital birth, try to become acquainted with the routine practices there. Tell the obstetrician you see for your pre-natal checkups what you would like and what you hope to avoid. Find out what is likely to be allowed and what will almost certainly be refused. Get him to note what you want in your file. He will certainly be familiar with the alternative, more progressive attitudes to birth, and may be able to help you avoid some of the less essential routine procedures.

When you enter the hospital, enlist the support of one of the nurses on duty there. Even if she has read your notes, remind her of what has been agreed. You may be able to refuse an enema, if you really do not want one. If you are to be induced, ask why. If there is no real necessity, you may be able to avoid this as well. You may want to take your chances on tearing instead of undergoing routine episiotomy. You may also want the cord to be left to stop pulsing naturally before it is clamped and cut. But even if you are content to leave these procedures to the discretion of the hospital, do ask for your baby to be left with you for the first 30–60 minutes after the delivery – unless his survival seems to depend on his being removed for special care. And if you intend to breastfeed, make sure he is put in a crib by your bed instead of being taken to the nursery.

Here, your baby's father can play a valuable part. If he has prepared for the birth with you, he should be able to see that what has been agreed beforehand is respected by the staff.

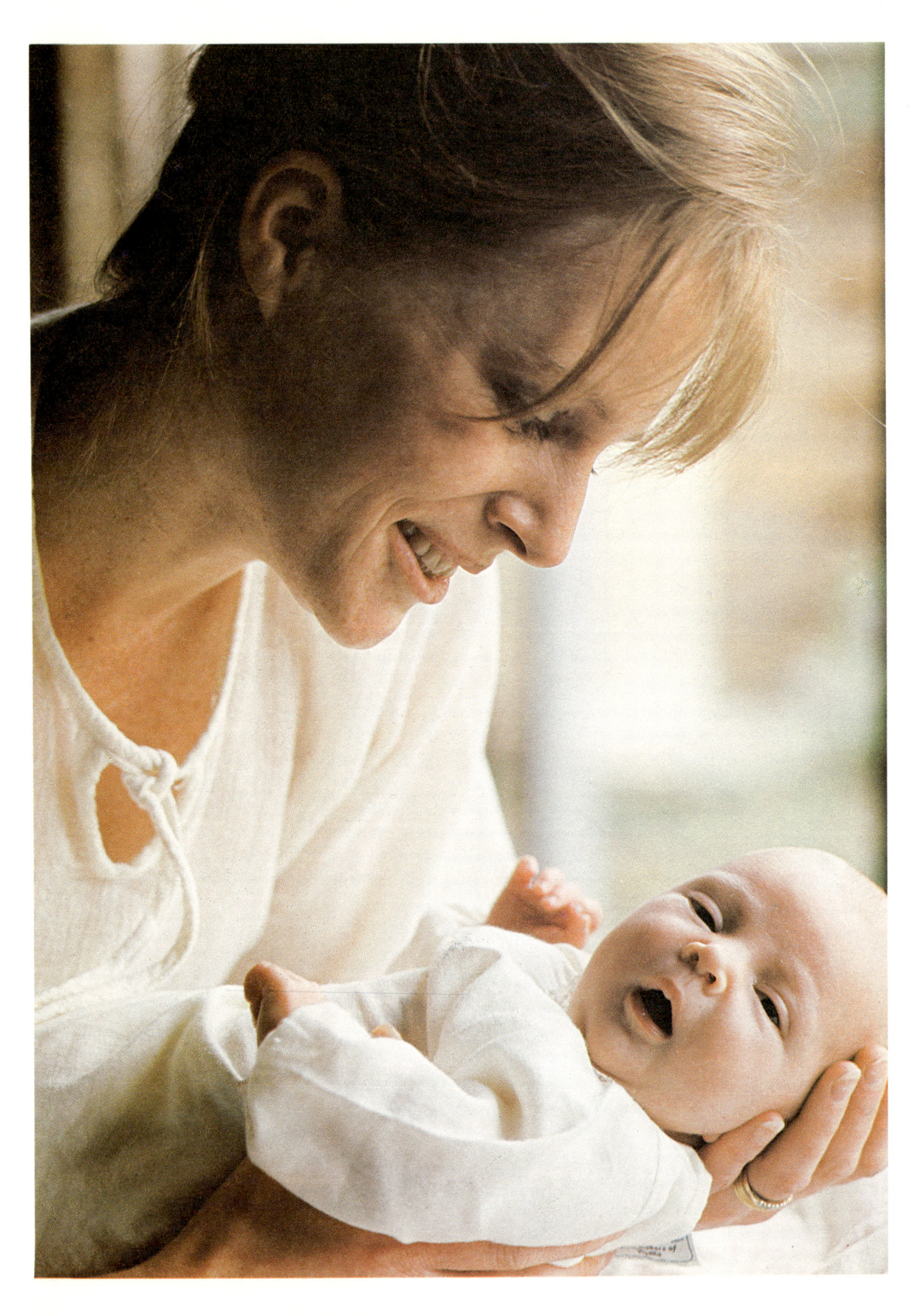

PART 2

Feeding the newborn

Your newborn child will have been through a tremendously exciting and perhaps frightening experience. More than anything else, he needs to be welcomed with love, to be reassured that all is well. If he is physically close to you, and you are at ease with him, he will quickly relax back into that blissfully calm state he knew in the womb. Then, you can rest together. Many babies are very alert for the first hour after birth and then sleep, perhaps with a few short interruptions, for a day or so.

During the pregnancy, your baby was of course fed continually through the umbilical cord. But now it is the mouth that receives his nourishment, so that a very special interaction develops between his mouth and your nipples, or the nipple of the bottle. Over the next few months, this feeding interaction will play a vital role, perhaps the key role, in your relationship with your baby, providing what are potentially your closest moments together. If these feeding times are harmonious, the chances are that your broader relationship will also be a harmonious and rewarding one.

Early feeding

Many babies take an early interest in feeding, happily sucking within hours or even minutes of birth. Because sucking on the breast stimulates the post-natal contractions of the uterus, helping restore it to its original size, this can also be beneficial to the mother. But do not worry if your baby seems not to want to suck at first, and do not wake him up to feed if he is happily asleep. If he grew to full term in the womb, his body will have stored up enough carbohydrate and fat to provide him with sufficient energy for a day or two following birth. Some babies are rather slow to begin, however, either because they are dulled by drugs that have been administered to the mother during labor (though they usually recover sufficiently by the second day to feed normally), or because they were born with some defect that makes sucking difficult for them. Down's Syndrome babies and those with cleft palates need particular assistance, though these infants can sometimes even be breastfed if the mother gets enough guidance and support.[6,7]

In many hospitals, sugar (or glucose) water is routinely supplied for a baby's first feeding, and also between feedings over the first few days. For babies who are to be bottle-fed, this provides a transition to a diet of full-strength formula. It may also be beneficial to a baby who has had a traumatic birth that has depleted his energy stores, if breast milk is not available. But sugar water is quite unsuitable for a healthy full-term baby who is to be breastfed. It encourages him to suck on the bottle when he should be using his energy to suck on the breast, which stimulates the mother's milk flow into full production. And it provides him with nothing but water and empty calories, instead of the highly nutritious, anti-infective first milk, known as *colostrum*. If breastfeeding, you can simply decline any offer by the hospital staff of sugar water, unless you are convinced that for some reason it is necessary.

Sucking and swallowing

Your newborn baby knows instinctively how to suck and swallow. In the womb, he will perhaps have sucked his thumb and he will certainly have swallowed a good deal of amniotic fluid, almost as if his digestive apparatus were preparing itself for the process of feeding after the birth. To get his sucking instincts going, however, you may need to show him where to start. An alert baby will often respond to a gentle stroking of his cheek by turning towards the sensation. If he finds a nipple or a bottle there, touching his lips, he will probably open his mouth to receive it in an automatic response. This is the *rooting reflex*. In breastfeeding, it triggers off the flow of milk from the breast, in a process that is known as the *let-down reflex*.

The amount of milk your baby drinks will depend on his needs at any particular time. Given as much as he wants, and provided that he is well and has recovered sufficiently from the effects of any drugs given to you in labor that may have entered his system, he will suck at the breast until he has had enough. As far as is known, there are two major influences on how much he will need to drink before this point is reached: one is his size, the other is the composition of the milk.

Heavier babies tend to need more by way of milk intake in order to maintain their larger tissue requirements; lighter ones tend to need less.[1] There are, however, certain exceptions to this. Premature babies, for instance, tend to continue to grow at the same rapid rate as in the womb, so they need, and get, more milk per pound of their weight than full-term babies.

The composition of your baby's milk – the balance of various nutrients in it – also has a direct influence on how much he will need to suck before he is satisfied.[2] He simply seems to adjust his sucking to match the composition of each feeding, stopping when his body has had enough. This adaptation of the baby to the milk is particularly important in breastfeeding, for breast milk varies quite naturally in composition from day to day, from feeding to feeding and from one part of a feeding to another. The first milk of each feeding is, for example, quite watery, providing a drink rather than food, and the baby sucks rapidly at this. As the feeding progresses, however, each breast yields an increasingly fat-rich milk, which the baby receives by sucking more slowly.[2] This matching of the baby's sucking to the milk is an instinctive two-way process, a part of the ongoing physical relationship between mother and baby. It also occurs in a 24-hour rhythm. Night feedings become richer in fat, thus shortening the time that has to be spent feeding.[3]

Patterns in feeding

In bottle-feeding, this adaptation of baby to mother and mother to baby is less marked, for the formula has a constant composition. The baby can, if allowed to drink when and as much as he wants, regulate how much formula he sucks. But if his sucking slows down at the end of a feeding of formula, he will not receive a richer milk: nor does he get a richer formula at night.

If a bottle-fed baby is fed by the clock, this biological matching of milk-intake to physical requirement can cease to function altogether.[4] His natural rhythms of hunger are subordinated entirely to the feeding pattern imposed by the parent or nurse. The baby tends simply to drink what he is given. This can sometimes be more than he actually needs – one reason why bottle-fed babies tend to grow faster, and fatter, than those who are breastfed.

Any tendency to over-rapid growth is also reinforced if the mother gives a bottle at those times when the baby cries for comfort, company, or reassurance, but is not really hungry for food. He wants to suck but not necessarily for a meal. This kind of 'feeding' is known as *non-nutritive sucking*. For a breastfed baby, non-nutritive sucking will usually yield very little milk, especially if the breast has not yet refilled after the last feed. But it does provide the reassurance of the breast, and it may also stimulate the baby to produce and swallow enzyme-rich saliva that aids digestion of an earlier meal.[5] In contrast, if the bottle-fed baby who needs to suck for comfort is offered a full bottle of milk, he will tend to drink. So try not to be too quick to give your baby a suck when he cries. If you are bottle-feeding, try holding and comforting your baby first.

Very small babies

Babies of low birth weight (LBW) often present feeding difficulties right from the start, while those weighing less than 3½ pounds, who are designated 'very low birth weight' (VLBW) normally need special care. LBW babies are often full-term but lighter than average. They can usually suck, although they may need frequent small feedings until their capacity for larger meals has developed. VLBW babies are generally born before term and need special attention.

VLBW babies pose special feeding problems because they are still growing at that very fast rate that normally occurs during the last two months in the womb. They need high concentrations of certain nutrients like iron, Vitamin E, and protein; and they need incubation and extra heat-generating food to keep them warm. There is much controversy among pediatricians as to the best milk for them. Had they remained in the womb, their umbilical food would have been very different from what is normally available in breast milk after the birth, and this has led some authorities to recommend a special formula. There is some evidence, however, that the milk of the mothers of VLBW babies adapts to the premature birth, supplying a richer concentration of certain nutrients than is normal for breast milk.[8,9] If this is the case, breast milk is the best choice, though it may need to be expressed and fed to the baby with a special bottle until he has matured sufficiently to suck well at his mother's breast. The pooled breast milk in hospital milk banks is generally considered unsuitable for VLBW babies because it is milk that comes from the mothers of full-term babies.[10]

VLBW babies are often too small and weak to suck, or tend to vomit up what they do suck. Their hunger can upset them so much that they fail to suck at all, and so they may have to be fed through a naso-gastric tube, which is passed through the nose straight into the stomach. But as soon as a tube-fed baby is able to suck at the breast or a small bottle, this form of feeding will be stopped.

If you do have a VLBW baby in special care and want him to be fed breast milk, you may be able to arrange to express it for him. Discuss this with the pediatrician and the nursing staff. If you are not incapacitated by caesarian section, spend as much time as you can in physical contact with your baby, and try to get him onto the breast as soon as possible. Once home, all being well, he will quickly start to gain weight.

Jaundice

Jaundice is common among both breast and bottle-fed babies during the first week of life, especially if they are born prematurely, but in almost all cases it lasts only a few days and presents no reason for a mother to stop breastfeeding her baby. The condition is recognized by a yellowing of the whites of the eyes and skin, due to a high level of *bilirubin* in the blood. Bilirubin is a breakdown product of old red blood cells. It is normally passed out of the body in bile, which is excreted in the feces; but in many newborn babies, the bile is retained in the blood.

According to the American physician Lawrence Gartner, the high blood bilirubin levels in neonatal jaundice are due to reabsorption into the blood of bilirubin from the baby's first feces – the thick, black *meconium* – for as long as the meconium sits in the bowel. He recommends breast milk *colostrum* as the best laxative to get the meconium moving, and points out that any other form of feeding may not only delay this first bowel movement but also leave the baby less interested in the breast. He argues strongly against the common hospital practice of giving babies sugar water and of recommending that formula-feeding should replace breastfeeding as a matter of course in cases of jaundice.[11]

Some breastfed babies develop another form of jaundice during their first week, and this can last for a month or more. Like the earlier form (known as *physiological* or *normal jaundice*), this *breast milk jaundice* presents no reason for a mother to stop nursing. Exposing the baby to daylight (not strong sunlight which could burn him) will reduce the bilirubin level. In the hospital, this may be done with *phototherapy*, a form of treatment which involves exposure to special fluorescent lighting. Sometimes Vitamin E injections are also given in an attempt to speed up the baby's recovery from the jaundice.[12]

At the breast

If this is the first time you have breastfed, you may be a bit bewildered by the prospect. Quite naturally, you will want to know when your baby is hungry, how to hold him, when you may need to burp him, when to switch breasts, and so on. Any sensitive, experienced nurse or another breastfeeding mother will be able to help you, but remember that the feeding experience is basically between you and your baby. If he is close to you from the start, you will quickly learn what he wants and how best to give it to him.

You will want to nurse your baby in a comfortable position. Some mothers prefer to nurse in bed, either lying down or propped up with a few pillows: others prefer to sit in a chair. Earlier in this century, it was quite easy to find nursing chairs, especially designed with low arms and an upright back to fit the nursing mother's requirements. Few are made today, but you should find that secondhand ones are still available. You need to be absolutely comfortable so that you can relax: tension, physical or mental, is a major obstacle to successful lactation.

In the first few minutes of feeding, the milk may rush out, forcing the baby to gulp and to swallow a lot of air. If your baby seems to have difficulty coping with this rush, let him suck a little, then gently release the nipple and take a short rest before continuing to feed again. Keep repeating this procedure, changing breast from time to time until the flow of milk slows down and your baby can suck in a more relaxed manner.

If your baby seems to be sucking only weakly, check that his mouth is properly fixed over the nipple, enclosing it completely. You may have to help him with this at first. Poor sucking can sometimes be due to lethargy, brought on by being too warmly covered. If you think this may be the case, uncover his feet, and perhaps play with them. Tease him with the nipple and put a few drops of milk on his lip. If your breasts are uncomfortably full, express a little milk into a cup or while you are having a bath. This will help you feel more comfortable.

Fixing the baby's mouth onto your nipple may also prove difficult if he is too excited, which may occur regularly during your early feedings. See that the flesh of your breast is not obstructing his nose; you may have to hold it back with your free hand. Also check his nostrils. During the first day or two, they may be blocked by mucus, which you can sometimes squeeze out gently between your thumb and forefinger. Once satisfied that he can breathe easily, you can adopt quite a passive role if he fusses. In general, the calmer and quieter your environment, and for some babies the dimmer the light, the quicker they settle down during a feeding. This can be especially important for babies who have had a difficult birth. Feeding times need to be as relaxed as possible.

Try to make sure that your baby is at each breast for an equivalent time, and begin each feeding with alternate breasts. As the breast milk composition changes quite normally from the beginning to the end of each feeding, this will ensure that he gets a balanced diet. It will also prevent your breasts from filling unequally with milk, which can be uncomfortable. To prevent the unsuckled nipple from dripping, while your baby is at the other breast, press against it with your free forearm.

There is no need to restrict your first feedings to one minute at each breast, increasing this by one minute with successive feedings, as is sometimes recommended, unless this coincides with your own feelings. Recent research at the Queen Charlotte Maternity Hospital in London has shown that babies breastfed in this strict way are less likely still to be breastfed a month later than babies who were fed according to their own unique requirements and rhythms. The same applies to the famous four-hour feeding system, which is still recommended for convenience in many hospitals. This was an idea that was introduced for bottle-feeding: it can only have a disruptive effect on lactation.

Breastfeeding by the clock is bound to be a struggle because full breasts cannot wait to be emptied, even if hungry babies can be made to wait. The Committee on Nutrition of the American Academy of Pediatrics has recognized this and now recommends demand-feeding in all hospitals.[2] If you allow your baby to indicate when and how much he should be fed during the early weeks, you will both fall easily into a shared rhythm.

If you have had a traumatic delivery, perhaps a caesarian section, you may be advised to bottle-feed. A combination of pain, exhaustion and an inability to move about may well tend to make you agree, even if you had originally planned to breastfeed. Yet, with help, you could probably make a start with breastfeeding right away. And once started, the very act of nursing may itself help you to get over any disappointment at not having had a normal birth. It may also speed up your recovery. After a caesarian section, breastfeeding has the additional advantage of stimulating the uterus to contract, which in turn revitalizes the abdomen. If you cannot move about easily, try feeding your baby lying down on your side. To change breasts, put him on your chest and slowly roll over to the other side. Determination and good spirits, plus the help of your baby's father and if possible the advice of another breastfeeding mother, will soon see you back to good health.

At the breast

Breast care

Breastfeeding is usually an enjoyable experience, but it can be irritating or even a little painful at times. If, however, you attend well to your breasts and nipples during these early weeks, you can prevent many unnecessary problems.

When feeding, let your baby suck as much as you comfortably can, gradually increasing the time as you adjust to each other. But take care not to continue too long, or your nipples may become sore. At the end of the feeding, if you need to release the vacuum-like grip of your baby's mouth, press on the breast close to the nipple but do not try to pull the nipple out of his closed mouth or you may hurt the nipple. After feeding, your breasts will normally be fairly empty. You can gently express any remaining milk if you feel uncomfortable, but this will not usually be necessary. Regular feeding is the best insurance against blockage of the milk ducts and infection.

Engorgement is a common problem due to a build-up of blood and milk. It can be eased, as here, with a cold, damp cloth.

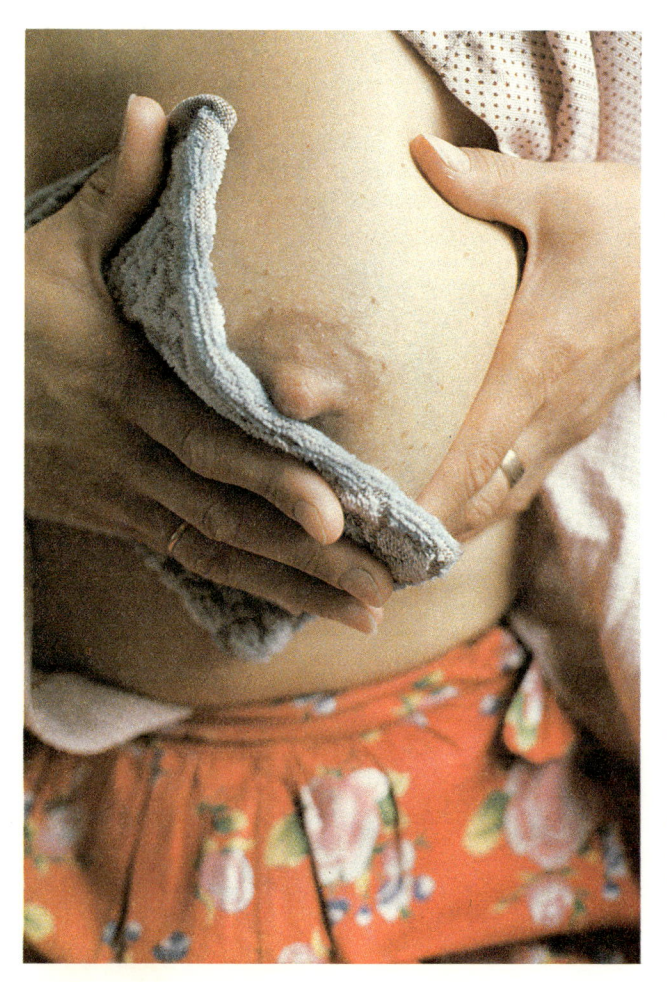

SORE NIPPLES can occur at any time if they have been roughly treated or left moist for too long. They may become inflamed and, if untended, the skin may crack. If you can, keep feeding or the milk ducts are likely to become blocked and your breasts may become engorged. Expose your nipples to air and sunlight as much as you can (but watch out for sunburn!), and keep them oiled with edible vegetable or Vitamin E oil, which the baby can safely suck, providing he is not put off by the smell.

ENGORGEMENT, a painful swelling of the breasts, is a common early problem, due to excessive fluid pressure in the breasts. In the first weeks of feeding, it is usually caused by a build-up of blood as the breast tissue awakens to its task of feeding. Later, engorgement is usually due to the pressure of unsucked milk. The breasts feel heavy, hot and tender; the armpit glands may be swollen, and sometimes there is fever. Because engorged breasts make feeding very painful, sometimes even impossible, act as soon as you realize what is happening and try one of the following treatments.
Heat treatment Soak the breasts in warm water until the pressure subsides; then massage to express some milk. You can do all this while relaxing in the bath.
Cold treatment Hold a cold, damp cloth to the breasts, recooling it as necessary, until the swelling is reduced.

MASTITIS is an inflammation of the breast usually resulting from a blockage of milk left to accumulate in the ducts. It can lead to infection. The warning sign is a sensitive pink spot on the breast, followed by a feverish feeling and pain when feeding. The best treatment is to keep on feeding as your baby's sucking will actually ease the blockage. Offer the good breast first and, as the milk starts to flow, massage the inflamed breast gently from the tender spot towards the nipple. This can be intensely painful at first, but the discomfort will ease as the milk block disperses. Between feedings, it may be helpful to splash the breasts alternately with hot and cold water, ending with cold. If infection develops and you have to take antibiotics, you *can* keep on feeding. The baby may develop a passing rash or another mild allergic reaction to the drugs, but this should quickly pass.

More about breastfeeding

The first few weeks may be rather trying as you and your baby get to know each other and establish a mutually acceptable feeding rhythm. At first, nursing every two or three hours is common, with a decrease to approximately four-hour intervals over the first month, but there are no hard and fast rules. Once settled, this rhythm may occasionally be disturbed by illness or major household changes – trips out for the day or house guests, for example – but it will probably hold fairly constant for the duration of breastfeeding. And breastfeeding is such a mobile affair that you should be able to stick to the rhythm almost anywhere. When you are out, find a quiet place to sit down and discreetly nurse. During recent years, many public places have come to accept the presence of a nursing mother, so that nowadays you are far less likely to be banished to the bathroom than was once commonly the case.[1]

The breastfeeding experience

Imagine your baby is now two months old and he starts crying in that way which you know means hunger: gently at first, then more vigorously. From experience, you know it is best to stop whatever you are doing and prepare yourself for feeding. You make yourself comfortable with him, perhaps with a drink by your side. Breast milk is mostly water, so you have to drink more fluids than usual. He may start to suck straight away or, if he is very hungry and excited, play about for a while before he sucks. All you need to do is relax, perhaps breathing deeply a few times: the milk will come. Try to find a quiet environment. While some babies suck in the midst of noise and bustle, interruptions sometimes disturb the milk flow.

During his feeding, your baby may stop to rest or play with you again for a while. If the first breast is fairly well emptied, you can take the opportunity to help him bring up any wind before switching to the other breast. This is burping. Put him against your shoulder and gently press against his lower back, stroking or patting to release any swallowed air. Don't slap him heartily on the back: he might bring up part of his feed if you do. After the second breast, you can always return to the first one if he seems to need more.

If your baby goes to sleep leaving your breasts uncomfortably full, you can rouse him by gently moving the nipple against his mouth, stroking his throat and lower jaw, or moving one of his arms towards his head. A baby who repeatedly falls asleep without having nursed completely is probably ill.

Expressing milk

Expressing milk – either because your breasts are overfull, or to provide a bottle-feeding for your baby while you are separated for some reason – may be done by hand or with a special vacuum pump. When expressing by hand, your fingers replace the baby's sucking with gentle massage and squeezing. Massaging the breast towards the nipple promotes the flow of milk along the ducts, while gently squeezing and rotating the areola sends milk squirting from the nipple. Express milk from one breast until the flow slows down, then switch to the other. Before going back to the first again – there will now be more milk in it – gently massage it to stimulate the flow, then express a second batch. You should find you can normally express three times from each breast. Collect the milk in any sterile container that has a secure lid. A bottle or a sterile bag that fits into a bottle are ideal. All you need to do is put the sealed container of milk in the refrigerator. It will stay fresh for several days.

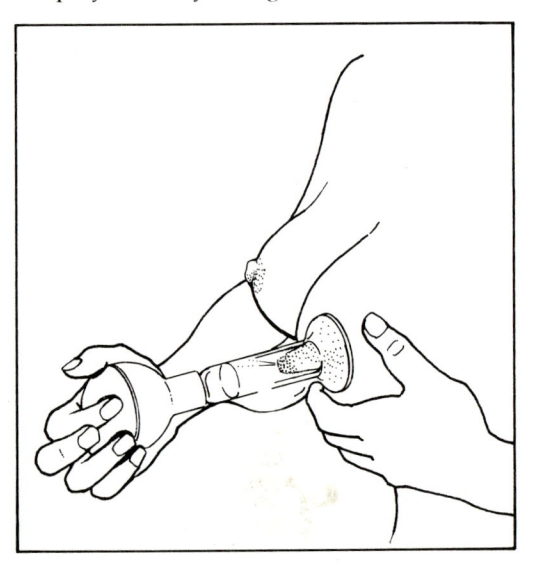

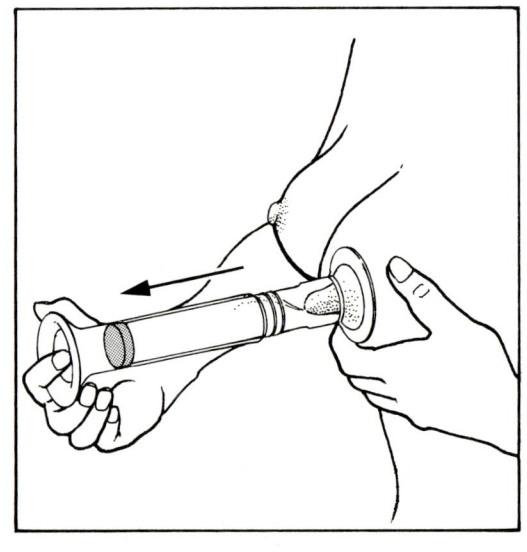

Milk can be expressed by hand or, as here, with a breast pump. Depress the flexible bulb to create a vacuum, fit it over the nipple, and release the bulb.

Breastfeeding an adopted baby

It is sometimes possible for a woman to breastfeed a small baby she has adopted by using a nursing supplementer to induce her milk supply. This consists of a sterile bag which delivers formula through a very fine, flexible tube into the baby's mouth as the baby sucks on the breast. Over a period of several weeks, this procedure induces lactation while the baby is fed at first through the tube, and later by a mixture of milk from the breast and formula delivered in the tube. Studies indicate that 50–75 percent of the adopted baby's food requirements can be supplied by breast milk once lactation has started. Peak milk production is reached after about twelve weeks. This procedure takes a good deal of faith, self-confidence and time, but can enormously enhance a mother's relationship with her adopted baby, as well as providing for the infant all the protective benefits of breast milk.[2]

How long should you breastfeed?

There are many reports of babies thriving on a diet of nothing but breast milk for over a year, with weaning taking place only gradually over the second, third, and even fourth year. However, the mother has to be healthy, well-nourished and, in our society, unusually dedicated. Most authorities in the United States and Europe recommend breastfeeding for a minimum of four–six months, and if feeding is going well, we strongly recommend that you do not offer your baby other foods until at least then. As we shall see, weaning is ideally a natural development over many months, a gradual process in emotional and physical development, not something you do to your baby over the course of a week.

If during the first six months you have to stop breastfeeding, perhaps to return to work, consider the possibility of expressing milk to be fed to the baby while you are away. If you do not have to stop, and would like to continue but feel exhausted, then take to your bed as if you were ill, and rest. Extreme tiredness can affect feeding. If you do decide to stop, however, do it as gradually as you can, cutting out feedings one at a time. The more gradual the transition, the easier it will be for you and your baby. Babies less than six months old should be switched to a formula: unmodified cows' milk is not suitable for babies at such a young age.

Do breastfed babies need supplements?

Once, most nutritionists would have answered 'yes' to the question of whether breastfed babies need supplements. Even as recently as 1978, Professor Samuel Fomon of the University of Iowa, for many years one of the most influential voices in the field of infant-feeding, wrote in the prestigious *New England Journal of Medicine*: "Human milk is unquestionably a superb food for infants. However, notwithstanding exuberant testimonials to the advantages of breastfeeding, human milk is neither a perfect nor a complete food."[3] There is, however, a vast body of evidence affirming the contrary. The breast milk of a healthy, well-nourished mother can be, and most commonly *is*, a perfect, complete food for her infant. How could the human race have evolved if it were not such a good form of nourishment? Mothers have been successfully breastfeeding their babies for millions of years. How, if a baby's fundamental food is not perfect (remember that there were no formulas until this century), could we all have survived to be healthy adults?

So in what nutrients was breast milk once considered lacking? One was iron. For many years breast milk was thought to contain very little iron and supplements were considered essential. Then it was discovered that the iron that there is in breast milk is bound up in a protein complex (*lactoferrin*), which is particularly well absorbed by the baby. The milk of a well-nourished mother who is breastfeeding without difficulty is now known to contain enough iron to satisfy the needs of a baby for as long as that milk is his whole diet, and this is true even to the end of the first year of life.[4]

Another stronghold of the 'breast milk is not adequate' school of thought was the belief that human milk contains no Vitamin D. This was based on the assumption that Vitamin D is *always* to be found in association with fatty tissue (it usually is) and, as there is no Vitamin D in breast milk *fat*, it was assumed there was none at all in breast *milk*. No one thought to look for the presence of this vitamin in the watery part of the milk. Vitamin D supplements were therefore considered to be essential for breastfed babies: and it was not until the 1970s that the presence of Vitamin D Sulphate was finally discovered in the watery part of breast milk.[5] Nature turned out to be not so imperfect after all!

The breast milk of a well-nourished mother is usually now considered to be a complete food for her baby for at least the first six months of life. Supplements are required by the baby only in those comparatively rare cases in which a mother has become so deficient in nutrients that her milk is also deficient as a result of her poor diet. In this situation, it is normally preferable to give supplements to the mother so as to improve the baby's diet by virtue of the milk composition, rather than to give any supplements directly to the baby.

The diet and breastfeeding

There is a new baby in the house, a source of joy and yet concern; an endless cause of repetitious tasks that fill your days and nights. There seems to be hardly a moment to think about yourself, let alone your diet. Yet, if you are breastfeeding, what you eat continues to be important, not only to keep *you* fit for the job but also – because your diet will affect your milk – to keep your *baby* well.

Our guidelines for a balanced diet in lactation are exactly the same as those for pregnancy. What you eat should remain a broad range of fresh unrefined foods. Do not worry that a few cakes, ice creams or hamburgers with ketchup are going to ruin breastfeeding. On the contrary, at this stage, if this is really what you feel like eating, and if it helps you relax and recover your sense of equilibrium, then it is almost certainly good for you. But as soon as you can, try to return to a balanced diet. If these processed foods are not what you want, however, get someone to bring in what you would like. Remember, too, that staying in bed can make you constipated, so try to get plenty of dried and fresh fruit, and wholewheat bread. But if like many women, you do not feel like eating much immediately after the birth, be sure not to let anyone bully you into it. Unwanted meals tend not to be digested very well.

How breast milk is made

Milk is produced in direct response to the baby. When he sucks on the nipple (and after a few weeks, even when he cries), nerve impulses flash rapidly from your breast to your brain. The brain responds by sending hormones to the *alveoli*, where milk is produced, and to the muscles round the alveoli. As the breast muscles contract, milk is secreted – via the ductules and ducts – to the nipple. The baby's sucking also helps to draw the milk down the ducts. The nipple, meanwhile, is lubricated by fluids secreted from the *Montgomery's tubercles*, situated in the areola, which become enlarged during lactation.

The first milk that comes into your breasts is a yellowish fluid called *colostrum*. It contains some fat and carbohydrate, as well as vitamins and minerals; but perhaps more importantly, it is rich in *immunoglobulins* (immunity proteins) that immunize your baby against certain diseases, including infection by the micro-organisms *E Coli* and *shigella*, common causes of infant diarrhea, and – if the mother has received polio vaccine – against polio.[1] During the first week, the colostrum is gradually replaced by an increasingly bluish milk containing rather less protein but more carbohydrate and fat: and the composition continues to change until, towards the end of the second week, the milk is said to be 'mature'. By then, it has half the original protein content, significantly more fat and carbohydrate, and a lower level of vitamins and minerals than colostrum. These changes are genetically programmed and almost certainly geared very closely to the changing nutritional needs of your newborn baby.

There is a good deal of variation between the milk of any two mothers and, as we have seen, in the milk of any one mother from morning to evening. In this respect, milk is like blood, which varies according to many aspects of the mother's life. As milk is produced in the breasts by nutrients that are carried there via the blood, the natural rhythmic fluctuations in milk and blood content are probably related to each other. And because the nature of your diet has a direct influence upon your blood, so it also influences your milk.

Theoretically, you need to eat more than you did during pregnancy, to provide for the milk; for during breastfeeding your body is putting out about six hundred more calories per day than usual, perhaps a third of the energy a mother receives from her food.[2] This does *not* mean that you have to eat another six hundred calories of food per day, however. Part of the energy for breast milk has been stored up in fat and muscle during pregnancy, and this extra weight gradually melts away as the months of feeding pass. Only part of the energy for feeding will come from your diet. As in pregnancy, nature arranges the delicate balance of needs and supply by adjusting your

The baby sucks, the mother responds. Breastfeeding provides all the food and the physical contact your baby needs.

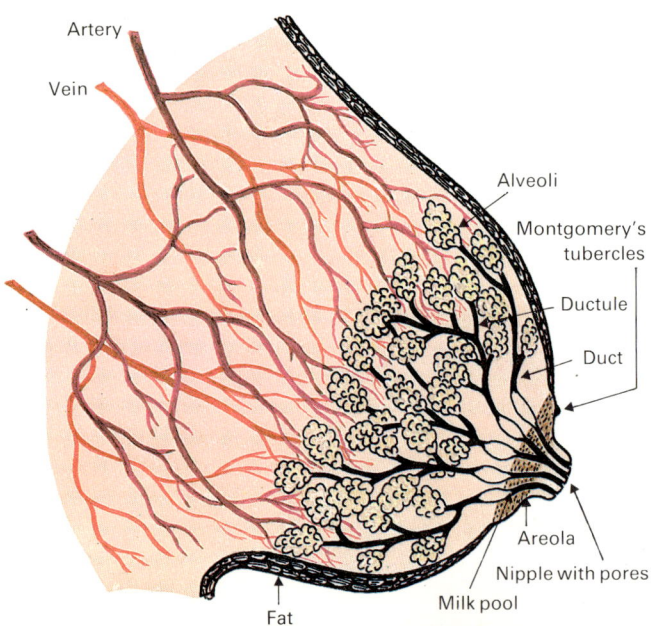

Artery
Vein
Alveoli
Montgomery's tubercles
Ductule
Duct
Areola
Nipple with pores
Milk pool
Fat

The diet and breastfeeding

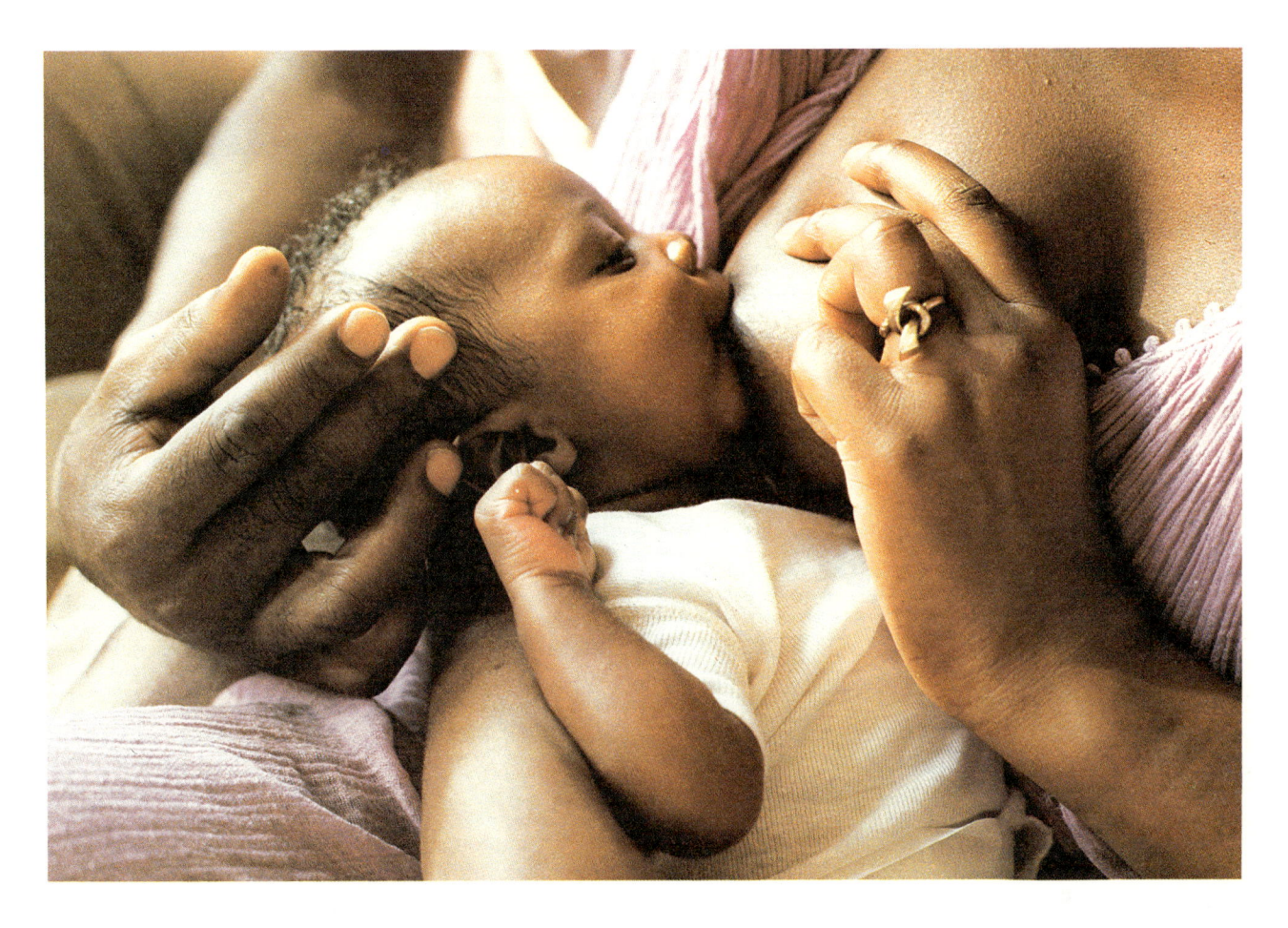

appetite. Rather than eating an extra six hundred calories a day, simply because you feel you ought to do so, trust your appetite. If you started doing this before the birth, it will come quite easily now. You may well feel like eating more than usual, and that is fine. But if you barely notice a change in your appetite, trust that, too. Appetite is a far more reliable guide than any theoretical extra.

The breastfeeding mother's diet is more important to the *quality* of her milk than to the *quantity*, because the nutrients that make up the bulk of the milk (proteins, fats and carbohydrates) tend to be taken from the mother's body stores, even if she eats a poor diet. Only if you are severely malnourished is the quantity reduced. But the quality of the milk – especially the vitamin concentration – *does* depend on your diet: in particular, the milk concentrations of certain B-vitamins and also Vitamin C are in direct proportion to the amounts of these vitamins in your food intake.[3] Your diet during breastfeeding therefore remains important.

In fact, anything you take into your body can come through into the milk and harm your baby. So, just as during pregnancy, try to avoid taking any drugs: and if you smoke, keep it to an absolute minimum. If your doctor prescribes drugs

Breast milk and love: natural nourishment for body and mind, and a complete diet for at least the first six months.

at any time, you may have to stop breastfeeding until their effects wear off. He or she will advise you on this. If you do stop for a while, keep expressing your milk, even if you have to throw it away, in order to keep the milk production going. If you do not do so, your milk may dry up.

But what of the actual composition of the breast milk? What does it contain that makes it so beneficial for a baby?

Approximately seven percent of breast milk consists of *lactose*, the milk carbohydrate. Together with much smaller amounts of other carbohydrates, lactose is very important to the establishment and maintenance of a colony of bacteria in the newborn infant's bowel. This colony is essential to the baby's defence system against foreign, disease-forming bacteria. One of the protective bowel bacteria, *lactobacillus bifidus*, is a deterrent against those bacteria that cause infant diarrhea, and it is the breast milk carbohydrates that promote its growth.[4] The lactose content of the milk seems to be independent of the mother's diet.

The diet and breastfeeding

Breast milk also contains between three and four percent fat, including a certain amount of *cholesterol*. Though eating too much cholesterol is believed to contribute to heart disease, we humans normally synthesize small amounts which we need for healthy nerve tissue and bile. It seems, too that babies probably need *some* dietary cholesterol for the development of enzymes that are necessary to metabolize dietary cholesterol after weaning.[5] It may also be that adults who were bottle-fed are more prone to high blood cholesterol levels. A current study that is being carried out in the Boston area which seems to support this view shows that thirty-year-olds who, as babies, were exclusively breastfed for more than two months have significantly lower blood cholesterol levels in adult life than those of the same age who were not breastfed in this way.

The amount of fat in the milk varies according to a number of factors including diet, ethnic origins, and 24-hour diurnal rhythms. Mothers who eat a low-fat diet, for instance, tend to give a milk containing slightly less fat than that of mothers whose consumption of fat is greater. The milk of all mothers also tends to be richer in fat at night than it is during the day.[6] In the West, we tend to eat more fat than is normal in poorer countries and our milk tends to be richer in its nutritional value, although there is no demonstrated advantage in this.

Breast milk contains surprisingly little protein: approximately two percent in colostrum (the first breast milk), much of it in the form of *immunoglobulins*, and less than one percent in mature milk. The transfer of immunoglobulins, which started via the umbilical cord in late pregnancy, drops off about two days after birth, but is later reinforced if the baby *does* develop an infection. In this case, the infection seems to be transferred from the baby to the breasts during feeding; and antibodies, produced by the mother, are returned to the baby in the milk.

The amino-acid pattern of breast milk protein is particularly suited to the metabolism of the human baby and is quite different from the pattern of cows' milk proteins. This is one reason why so many bottle-fed babies have an allergic reaction to cows' milk. However, the total protein content of your mature milk remains relatively unchanged regardless of your diet, though additional protein-rich foods (animal foods or grain-legume mixtures) may increase it slightly if your diet has been *very* poor. Similarly, extra protein can increase the quantity of milk if a mother's normal diet is very low in protein. But for well-nourished women, protein supplements do not improve either milk quality or quantity. If, therefore, your diet is well balanced, protein supplements will not be necessary during the time you are breastfeeding.

Vitamins in breast milk

The concentration of many of the vitamins in your milk is known to be directly related to the amounts of these nutrients in your food.[7] To what extent low intake of any of these nutrients, and hence low levels in the milk, can affect the baby will depend largely on your baby's stores at birth. For example, a mother who ate very few *thiamin* (B_1) rich foods in pregnancy – whole grains, meat, beans, nuts, and dark green leafy vegetables – will probably give birth to a baby with low thiamin stores. If her diet remains low in thiamin and she breastfeeds, the baby will become B_1-deficient, developing the infantile neuro-muscular disease *beriberi* during the first few months. This condition is rare in the West but frequent in South-East Asia, where low thiamin rice diets are common. Similarly, strict vegan mothers who took neither animal foods nor Vitamin B_{12} supplements during pregnancy are likely to give birth to babies with low B_{12} stores and a propensity for B_{12} deficiency (*pernicious anemia*), for Vitamin B_{12} is found only in animal products and a few herbs, like comfrey. If you took B_{12} supplements during pregnancy, you should continue to take them regularly throughout breastfeeding.

Vitamin A deficiency is common in the malnourished Third World, and is also reported among women in the West. In lactation, such deficiency may affect the vitamin content of your milk, so do include a range of Vitamin A-rich foods (like melon, sweet potatoes, butter, cabbage, and apricots) in your diet, so that the baby does not in turn become deficient.

The Vitamin C content of milk is highly dependent on the mother's current diet, while the baby's actual requirement for it will depend on the diet during pregnancy. If you took large doses of Vitamin C before the birth (1 gram per day or more), your baby may have been born with a higher than normal requirement, and may need a higher than normal Vitamin C content in his milk. This could mean that you should continue the supplements for as long as you breastfeed or the baby may become deficient in Vitamin C. We suggest you consult your doctor about this matter and the level of supplementation you need.

A mother's Vitamin D status may also affect her milk. If she is deficient, her milk will also be deficient and her baby's health may be affected. Rickets, with its characteristic bowing of the long bones, can result. The Roman physician Soranus described infant rickets in the second century, but believed it was due to inattentive mothers who had forced their babies to walk too soon.[8] More recently, it has been found among the breastfed babies of Arab women, whose diet is poor in Vitamin D, and whose veils and robes hide their skin from the sun. Skin, you may remember, produces its own Vitamin D on the action of sunlight.

The relationship between Vitamin D and the sun is an interesting one. Those whose skin is genetically adapted to the sun – black and certain Asian races, for example – appear to need more than white people. This can create problems for those who emigrate to cooler, darker environments, where there is less sunlight, for they now need to add additional Vitamin D-rich foods to their diet, though they may not be aware of this. Cod-liver oil, fish, eggs, lard, and Vitamin D-enriched milk and margarine are especially useful to them. Asians who settle in Britain, and Blacks in the United States, are among those who may be at risk.[9,10]

Minerals and milk

Less is known of the relationship between the mineral content of the mother's diet and the composition of her milk. With the exception of iodine, and possibly magnesium and zinc, all the evidence so far points to very little connection between the two.[11] Iodine is lacking from the diet only in areas where the soil – and therefore the food grown in it – is iodine-deficient, in which case iodized salt should be used. Magnesium and zinc are adequately supplied by a wholefood diet.

A mother's intake of calcium appears to have absolutely no effect on her milk composition.[12] To what extent this implies that her body will direct calcium from the bones and teeth for the milk if her dietary intake of calcium is low remains unclear. There is evidence that a breastfeeding mother, eating very few calcium-rich foods (milk, cheese, dark green leafy vegetables, nuts and seeds), may lose calcium from her bones to provide for her milk. However, Third World studies suggest that mothers who are adapted to a low calcium intake can breastfeed several children over a number of years without becoming calcium deficient, probably because they absorb the small amount of calcium in their diet with high efficiency, and lose very little calcium in the urine.[13]

Similarly, the breastfeeding mother's intake of iron bears no direct relationship to the iron content of her milk. Even if her iron intake is very low, the milk iron level remains constant.[14] In view of the small amount of iron in breast milk, this is perhaps not surprising. Even a mother with very low iron stores, perhaps because of having lost a lot of blood (and therefore iron) in labor, will provide enough for milk. In addition, breast milk iron is well retained by the baby: five times better, in fact, than the iron used in a formula.[15] (Recent research also shows that the same is true of zinc.) This is widely believed to be due to its unique protein-bound structure, lactoferrin.

Isotope studies show that lactoferrin not only fulfills the baby's dietary iron requirement, but also plays a part in the life of the useful bacteria that live in the baby's bowel: bacteria that protect against foreign diarrhea-causing bacteria. Without lactoferrin, the gut bacteria become changed and less effective in their protective function. Professor Elsie Widdowson of the British Medical Research Council has suggested that the protective role of breast milk iron is more important than its dietary role, for young babies quite naturally excrete more iron in their stools than they take in their milk.[16] It would be interesting to know why it is that this happens.

Liquid intake

As in pregnancy, you will need to pay as much attention to what you drink as to what you eat. If you found herbal teas acceptable then, continue using them now. Infusions of fennel and anise have been recommended for centuries to promote the flow of breast milk.[17] Both caffeine and alcohol pass into the milk in small amounts, so the more of either that you drink, the greater the chance that your baby will be affected. Two or three cups of coffee, tea, or hot chocolate per day will probably do no harm, if you are used to them: but watch to see if there is any effect on your baby. Caffeine, remember, is a stimulant. Similarly, if you drink alcohol, an occasional evening brandy or a couple of glasses of wine is unlikely to have an adverse effect on your milk, although some babies do become a little drowsy for a while. But the more you drink, the more likely it is that you will make your baby ill and also reduce your milk flow at the same time.

Water – especially bottled or fresh spring water – is probably the best drink you can have. Breast milk is in fact largely water, so you need to drink to replace the losses. But do not drink out of duty! One study has shown that mothers who drank a *prescribed* six pints of water a day had a smaller milk supply than when they were drinking simply to quench a thirst. You really do need to follow your own body signals.

Vegetable soups are also good for you while breastfeeding, especially if made with potassium-rich vegetables, for potassium losses in the milk are relatively high. Zucchini, potatoes, spinach, artichokes, mushrooms, lima beans, butter beans and parsley are all suitable. Simply clean and cut up a mixture of any of these, sautée them lightly in a little oil, add plenty of water, turn down the heat, and simmer for twenty minutes. Add seasoning or a few chopped chives before serving. Other good sources of potassium are wheat germ, apricots, and figs.

Early bottle-feeding

Bottle-feeding with one of the modern formulas will provide your baby with a more or less balanced diet of the important nutrients and can – if you and your baby also have plenty of physical contact – be a warm and friendly experience for both of you.

If this is your first baby, you will probably need some help with bottle-feeding to start with, and the nurses at the hospital, or the midwife, should certainly be able to provide this for you. Every packet and tin of formula is labeled with detailed instructions, but they are not always easy to understand at first. You will soon get used to them, however. Most labels also contain a chart that tells you approximately how much to give your baby at each feeding, as well as how many feedings to give each day over the next few months. It is essential to follow these instructions for quantity closely.

Although hospital procedure is usually to feed all babies together at three or four hourly intervals, you can, if you wish, ask to have your baby by your bed in order to feed him yourself whenever he seems to be hungry. Feeding by the clock is more convenient to the hospital staff, of course, and many believe that fixing the times of a baby's meals from a very early age is a good idea because it 'gets them into regular eating habits'. In our experience, the reverse is true: feeding by the clock can run you into trouble. There is nothing more likely to give you a headache than the sound of your unhappy baby screaming with hunger while you wait for the fixed time of his feeding to come around. Nor is there anything more frustrating than to try to force a meal on him when he simply is not hungry. Eventually, like Pavlov's dogs who learned to salivate at the ring of a bell, your little one will become accustomed to eating on time, but the price could be high. If his sense of hunger is not respected now – so that he is fed when he is hungry, and only then – he may well develop eating disorders later. American researchers Wright and Fawcett have shown that whereas demand-fed babies establish a rhythm of feeding by the second month (which makes life much easier for everyone), those fed by the clock fail to find their own rhythm until after they are weaned, at about six months.[1] Another study has shown that babies fed on demand (when they are hungry rather than when their mothers require them to eat) are more likely to be of normal weight and confident enough to sustain separation for brief periods from their mothers than those babies whose hunger signals are ignored. The more you can accommodate yourself to your baby and his needs at the beginning, the easier things will be later on. For eating disorders among children and adults – in which the physiological regulations of hunger have broken down – can sometimes be traced back to very rigid feeding patterns begin back in early infancy.[2]

Demand-feeding is more trying for a bottle-feeding mother than for the mother who simply has to find a quiet spot and offer her breast, but it *is* worth the extra effort. If you go visiting with the baby, take a sterilized bottle containing the measured formula powder for a feeding, and a thermos flask of boiled water. Then, when your baby is hungry, simply add water to the bottle. To avoid the risk of contamination with bacteria, do not carry bottles of made-up formulas unless they are sealed and packed with ice: an insulated picnic box is suitable for this. Similarly, it is not a good idea to try to keep a bottle warm. Far better, warm the milk as it is required.

The formula

In the hospital, you will probably have been given one of the most recent brands of formula that are designed to resemble breast milk as closely as technology permits. Many hospitals buy their formulas already made up in small ready-to-feed bottles, but they are most commonly available in the stores as a powder that you have to make up into liquid feedings yourself. Instructions follow on page 60, and will also always be given on the packaging in which the formula comes.

Some babies are allergic to the cows' milk used in the standard formulas:[3] they develop eczema, breathing problems, or diarrhea if they drink it. If your baby does develop an allergic reaction to cows' milk while you are in the hospital, he will probably be offered a non-milk formula in its place. This may be based on soy instead of milk: but as soy allergy also occurs, there will be other soy-free, milk-free formulas available, too. If you have to use one of these special products at first, you need not worry that your baby will necessarily have a lifelong allergy. While this can be the case, the allergy is usually transient. Older babies generally take to ordinary cows' milk without difficulty.

If you give birth at home, and you intend to bottle-feed, arrange for a supply of formula to be available. It does not have to be one of the latest brands but it should be a product designed specifically for babies. This is something very important to remember. Ordinary unmodified cows' milk is not suitable during the first few months and could make your baby ill.

When you prepare your own formula, follow the mixing instructions very carefully. The relative quantities of powder and clean water must be carefully measured or the resulting milk is likely to be of the wrong strength, which may upset your baby. In general, nothing else needs to be

Early bottle-feeding

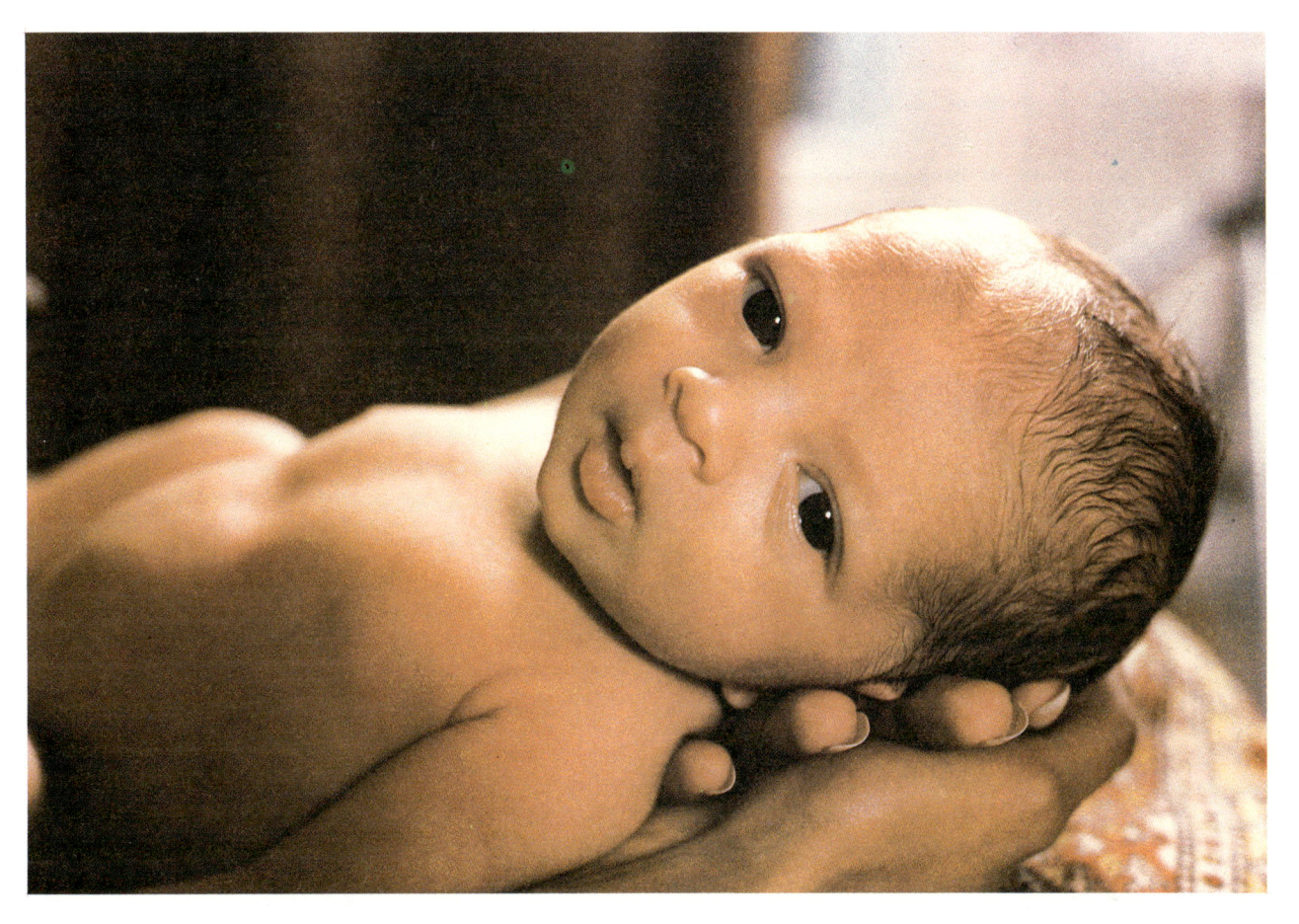

The breastfed baby gets a lot of physical contact. Bottle-fed babies need it even more.

added to the formula.

The actual quantity of made-up formula that you give your baby should depend on him. On the formula package or can are listed the average quantities a baby takes at each feeding, according to his age; but these are meant to be treated with flexibility. Some manufacturers add a note to this effect, pointing out that some babies will take more, some less. If you insist on your baby finishing a bottle when he has already taken enough, he will probably throw it up again within minutes. Conversely, if he seems to want another bottle, let him have it or he will fuss until he is satisfied. When the weather is hot, you might try offering a second bottle of boiled, cooled water: you can always go back to another bottle of formula if this does not satisfy him. In areas where the tap water is fluoridated, it may be a good idea to use non-carbonated bottled water instead. Fluoridated public water supplies clearly have an adverse effect on some babies, who tend to develop mottled teeth as a result.

To save time in preparing feedings, you can make them up in advance each day and store them in the refrigerator. Then, all you have to do when your baby is hungry is to warm a bottle. If for some reason you have no access to a refrigerator, nor any other very cool place, you will have to make up the bottles freshly each time. Bacteria breed easily in milk when it is not correctly stored. This can be unnerving when a baby is howling: but by stopping whatever else you are doing as soon as you hear his first call, you can avoid the worst of this.

It is important to pay attention to the size of the holes in the nipples you use. The holes should allow a stream of air bubbles into the bottle to replace the milk sucked out by the baby. If the holes are excessively large, too much air will get in, which your baby may swallow. This may give him heavy burps or stomach cramps. If the holes are too small, he will not be able to suck fast enough and may get very frustrated. In general, smaller babies need smaller holes in the nipples: larger babies need larger holes. Test, too, that the nipple holes are not blocked by shaking out a little of the content. Watch carefully to see how easily your baby seems to be feeding: and, if necessary, experiment with alternative nipples. You will always do well to have some nipples in reserve, in case they are needed.

Early bottle feeding

Mixing the formula

Mixing in a pitcher

1. Wash your hands. Boil the water. Use part to rinse out thoroughly both the baby bottle and a pitcher. Let the rest cool slightly.
2. Measure the required amount of warm, previously boiled water into the bottle. Then pour the water into the pitcher.
3. Add the required amount of formula powder into the pitcher with the scoop provided.
4. Mix the formula with a fork, spoon or whisk.
5. Pour the formula into the baby bottle. If you are making up several feedings at once, pour it into several bottles. Let the formula you are using immediately cool until comfortably warm.
6. Additional feedings must be stored in individual bottles with caps in a refrigerator and used within twenty-four hours. Before use, you can warm the formula by standing the bottle in hot water or use a special bottle-warmer. Shake the bottle before use.

Mixing in a bottle

1. Wash your hands. Boil the water. Use part of the water to rinse out the feeding bottle. Let the rest cool slightly.
2. Measure the required amount of warm, previously boiled water into the feeding bottle.
3. Add the required amount of formula powder with the scoop provided.
4. Place the cap on the bottle and shake gently.
5. Let the formula for immediate use cool until comfortably warm. Test its temperature by shaking a few drops on the inside of your wrist.

Reminders

1. Make up the feeding exactly as instructed on the packaging.
2. Never add more powder than indicated, even if you have been told that it will help the baby to sleep. It could make him very ill.

Emergency homemade formula

In an emergency, when breastfeeding is impossible and no modern formula is available, a baby can be fed with a homemade formula. Before the development of the modern formulas, half-strength cows' milk (and, in some countries, goats' and camels' milk) was commonly used for bottle-feeding, although they are far from ideal. The milk was diluted with thoroughly boiled water, reducing the protein and fat content to levels closer to those in breast milk, as was later discovered. Sugar would also be added to bring the carbohydrate level up to that of breast milk. Mothers were also advised to add a little *sodium citrate*, available in tablet form, or barley water to make the milk more easily digestible: this, it later turned out, also provided the baby with some protection against diarrhea. Instead of fresh whole milk, dried whole milk could also be used, reconstituted in the proportion of one part milk to seven parts water. If a baby *had* to be entirely bottle-fed on this formula, one ounce per feeding of sugar water (one part sugar to nineteen parts clean water) was recommended during the first few days.

The following recipe, based on the 1958 edition of Maggie Myles' *Textbook for Midwives*, will provide enough emergency formula for about twenty-four hours during the first eight weeks of a baby's life in case, for some reason, a commercial formula is not available. Careful preparation of the feeding is very important.

½ pint (1 large cup) whole cows' milk
½ pint (1 large cup) cool, boiled water
5 grams (1 tablet) sodium citrate, if available
2 level teaspoons sugar

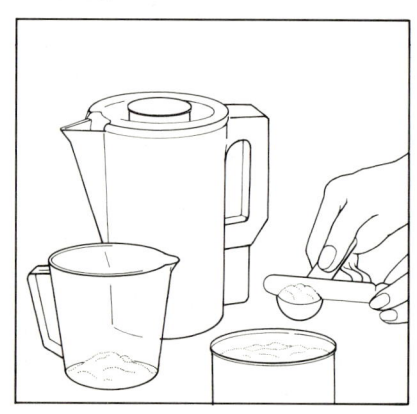

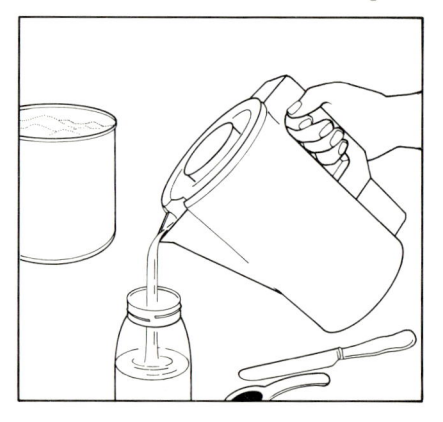

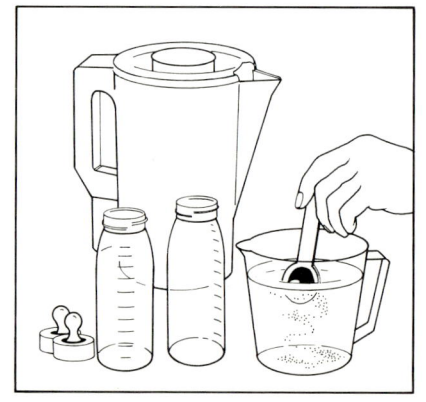

1. Pour the milk into a pitcher and ensure that the cream is mixed in.
2. Boil the water in a saucepan. Then add the milk to the water.
3. Bring milk and water to a boil, stirring constantly to prevent formation of a skin.
4. Boil milk and water for one minute, stirring constantly.
5. Remove from the heat.
6. Stir in the sugar.
7. Crush the citrate tablet finely and stir it in.
8. Pour the modified milk into five or six sterile bottles, if available.
9. Cover each one. Let them cool.
10. Store in a very cool place.
11. If the modified milk is kept in a pitcher, the milk must be stirred thoroughly.

If used into the third month, make up the emergency formula by diluting the half-pint of milk with only one quarter-pint (½ large cup) of water. This will give three-quarters strength milk for feeding. In the sixth month, it should be quite safe for you to give full-strength cows' milk without the need for added water.

Supplements when bottle-feeding

Before the development of the modern formulas, when modified cows' milk (as in the emergency homemade formula) was used, supplements of iron and Vitamins A, C, and D were required for all bottle-fed babies because there are not enough of these nutrients in non-human milks. These supplements can still be purchased, with a dropper for easy use, but are not required if you use a modern formula, which has all the known essential nutrients already added to it. And young babies are very sensitive to excess. During the 1950s, the British Department of Health recommended Vitamin D supplements at five times the dose recommended by the United States Department of Health. As a result, two hundred cases of Vitamin D overdosing were reported in Britain. Fortunately there were not more, apparently because many babies were able to excrete the excess in their feces. The recommended Vitamin D dose in the United Kingdom was subsequently reduced.[7] Today, few doctors would recommend such supplements for a baby receiving a modern formula.

Feeding with a bottle

Many babies accept bottle-feeding without difficulty, but they also need plenty of the physical contact that breastfed babies get quite naturally. Avoid treating your baby's feeding times as a task to be done quickly and efficiently. Relax with him and let him feel you, both during feedings and between them. Play with him. Bottle-fed babies are sometimes physically well-fed but emotionally starved.

Never leave the baby alone with a bottle of milk propped up in his mouth: he might choke. And, as he gets older, avoid putting sweet sugary drinks in the bottle. Bathing the teeth in a constant stream of sweet fluid is a sure way to encourage decay of newly erupting teeth, because it prevents the natural cleansing action of saliva on the teeth. Even fruit juice and milk can have this effect for as long as they remain in the baby's mouth, though it can take many months or even years for the decay to become apparent, depending on the natural strength of the teeth in the first place.

Changing the milk

It can be tempting in the early days of bottle-feeding to think that a change of formula will solve feeding problems. Sometimes a switch can be helpful: for example, a baby who cannot digest the fat in one brand may fare better with another. On the other hand, feeding problems can have many possible causes. But avoid changing more than twice: each brand has its own virtues and problems, and your baby is as likely to settle down with one as he is to fare better with yet another.

If you were unable to breastfeed during the first weeks and would like to start now, you may well be able to do so. The best stimulation for lactation is your baby's sucking, so offer him your breasts both between and during feeds. As long as your breasts have no milk, he may show little interest, although the use of a nursing supplementer, which delivers formula into his mouth through a fine tube which is stuck to your breast, may help. The baby sucks simultaneously on the breast and the tube, and receives both milk and formula at the same time. In this way, lactation is gradually induced. One of the breastfeeding organizations should be able to advise about this.

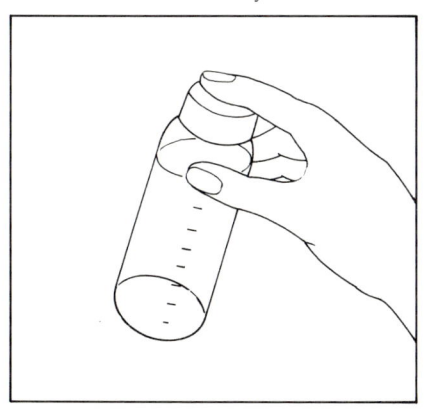

To make up a feeding in a pitcher, add the correct amount of powder to the cooled, boiled water and mix thoroughly. Fill the bottles and refrigerate. Alternatively, add the milk powder to a bottle of cooled boiled water and shake to mix the feeding.

The mother's well-being

You may well have been entranced by your baby during the first few days after the birth; but the ensuing weeks could turn out to be something of a sobering time, especially if this is your first child. The honeymoon is over: now you have to settle down to the immensely difficult, tiring and often lonely task of being a mother. Sometimes you will love it, sometimes you may feel driven to the limits of your sanity.

At first, your baby seems to have no sense of himself as someone separate from you or from the rest of the world. Everything simply 'is' in a world of dream-like impressions: lights and shapes, sounds from outside and inside his body, the touch of skin, of cloth, of water. Some impressions soothe him, some excite him, some frighten him. But none pleases and reassures him more than your presence.

Although it can be terribly frustrating to a mother to be needed so much, your baby's state of ease is very important to both of you, and to the rest of the household. For many women, the first few weeks involve a radical change of lifestyle. In some societies – in East Africa and India, for example – the first two months or so after the birth are treated as an incubation period, with the mother and her newborn closeted away together from the rest of the community, in order to give the two some time to adjust to their new relationship.

You were his entire old world for nine whole months; now you are the center of his new one. Only gradually over the first year does he come to see and accept that you and he are actually separate people.

Losing weight

As soon as your baby, and the placenta, are born, you will lose about ten pounds in weight. During the next few days, your uterus will periodically contract as it sheds the debris of tissue from the uterine walls. Together with fluid losses, you will quickly lose another five pounds or so.

During the next three months, most breastfeeding mothers lose another eight pounds or so which represents the fat and protein stores laid down in pregnancy, apparently to provide energy for lactation. Bottle-feeding mothers can lose the same amount of weight by a combination of careful eating and plenty of exercise to burn up fat stores. But whichever group you fall into, you will benefit by maintaining the balanced diet you established during pregnancy. Bottle-feeding mothers will, however, probably feel like eating a good deal less than breastfeeding mothers.

Breastfeeding mothers usually have a good appetite: and, because lactation is quite demanding, they may eat even more than in pregnancy. This is quite natural. If you can simply eat whenever you are hungry and stop when you have had enough, you will gradually lose the rest of that weight gained in pregnancy. Your body is 'programmed' to resume more or less its pre-conception state by the time lactation ends. Your milk quality does, however, call for a good daily intake of vitamins, with other nutrients coming from your body stores. And body stores themselves need to be replenished, so try to keep to a balanced diet as best you can.

Post-natal depression

Most women regain their pre-pregnancy weight, or something close to it, by the end of the first year, but about four in ten do not. Post-natal depression (PND), with a tendency to self-destructive eating habits, is one major cause. This is not the 'baby-blues' that mothers sometimes feel during the first few days after the birth, but a prolonged period of low-energy frustration and sadness over the first year. Typically, PND afflicts low-income mothers with several children who have had a hospital birth and are not breastfeeding. Many are also single parents.[1] Any one of a number of factors may bring on the depression. One mother has an episiotomy that fails to heal and finds herself unable to make love for a year. Another has a good delivery but finds the weight of duties at home too arduous and isolating. Tiredness during the early post-natal months, with their relentless day-and-night routines, is another major contributory factor. Battling against a downhill spiral of seemingly endless duties, lack of support and decreasing energy, many depressed mothers turn to the temporary consolation of desserts, candy, cookies and general overeating. Sadly, this only makes matters worse, not only by reducing available energy still more, but also by slowing down weight loss, which in turn tends to add to the depression.

Personal attention seems to be the most effective treatment of PND, but this is not always easy to find. Psychotherapy, hypnotherapy, co-counselling, group therapy – all can help, as may joining up with a local yoga, keep-fit or meditation group. And so can a balanced diet. If you find your eating habits running away with you, make up your mind to deal with the situation. This may seem appallingly difficult if food is your only comfort. One way to approach the problem is to eat nothing but raw food for twenty-four hours at least once a week. A day and night of uncooked vegetables, fruit, nuts, and seeds will refresh an overworked digestive system and revitalize the entire body. The change is usually noticed immediately.

The mother's well-being

Relieving the tension

Being a new mother (or father!) sometimes seems to be the hardest job on earth. You remember the times when you slept right through the night, every night, and wonder how you ever took them for granted. You struggle to carry the baby *and* the shopping, remembering how once there was only the shopping. You remember all the little things you used to like to do. If, at the same time, you are recovering from a tear you received as the baby was born, or an episiotomy, or even a caesarian section and all that involved, it can be a very tiring time.

You become tense, physically and mentally. Your muscles literally tighten up: it may be the arm you use to carry the baby; it may be your shoulders tensing up in response to yet another round of crying; it may be your back or your neck. You may become irritable, confused, even desperate. Yet there are many ways to keep this from getting the better of you. Following a post-natal exercise program is one method. We have run stretching and relaxation classes for mothers and babies: the mothers have a chance to stretch out their tight muscles (and tense minds) in a number of easy and beneficial exercises, while the babies are looked after in another room.

Night feedings will probably be the most inconvenient and exhausting part of it all. Some mothers adapt fairly easily and continue to night-feed throughout the first year. Others reach a point where they have to cut down on night feedings for their own health and sanity. If you feel this way, try to get your baby used to feeding just before you go to bed. This may forestall your having to get up an hour later. With a bit of luck, you might then only be disturbed once before dawn. Breastfeeding mothers are at an advantage because they do not need to prepare a bottle. On the other hand, some bottle-feeding mothers enjoy the advantage of a loving mate who can help them with this during the night, so that they can get the rest they need. Night feedings can be a very tiring business if you are bottle-feeding, so most mothers find.

Despite the vague assurances of the professionals that night feedings will be over within a few weeks of the birth, if you are well organized, you may find yourself still at it after several months. This can drive some women to the brink of breakdown. If you find yourself in this situation, get some help. You may just need a little time on your own to have a good sleep or to go for a walk. Have your mother or a friend look after the baby for a few hours. Or get in touch with your local branch of the La Leche League or a similar organization for new mothers. See page 96 for a list of useful addresses. Some may provide just the help you need at such times.

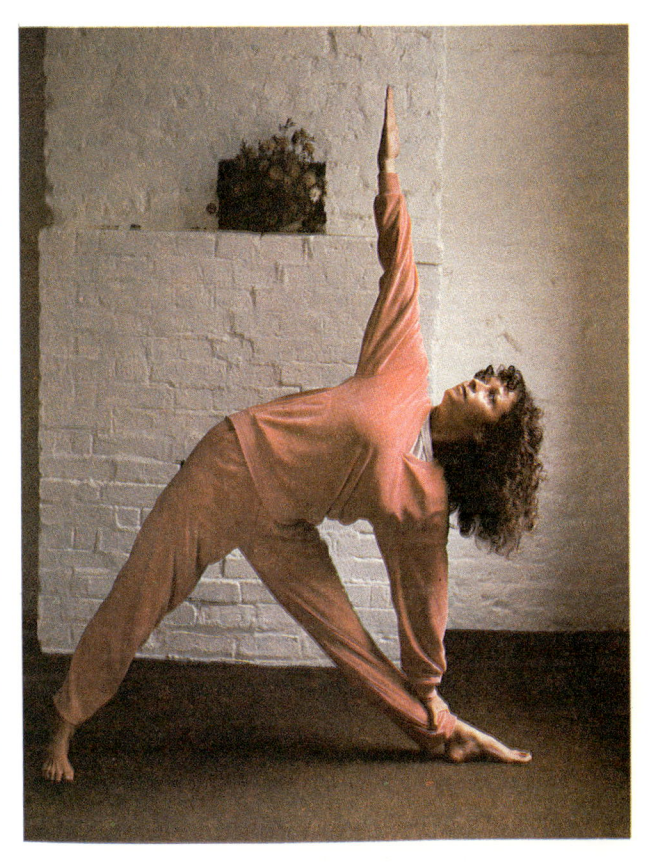

Post-natal yoga is a wonderful way to get back into shape.

Contraception

Although breastfeeding does offer some protection against conceiving another child – by suppressing ovulation – it is not a guarantee. Many breastfeeding women do not ovulate until lactation is over, but statistics suggest that one in three ovulates within four months of the birth: and from the time you start to replace breast milk with other foods – be it with a formula or semi-solids – your chance of ovulating within four weeks is two out of three.[2] So breastfeeding is clearly not the most reliable form of contraception. As if in recognition of this uncertain state of affairs, many traditional societies impose a taboo on lovemaking as long as the mother is nursing. If this approach appeals to you, there is no need to think about other forms of contraception at the moment. But if you do make love, and are not ready for another pregnancy yet, you need to be prepared. If you opt for the pill, be aware that some types can inhibit lactation. Seek your doctor's advice.

If you bottle-feed your baby, you may need to think about contraception right after the birth. Oral contraception can also increase a woman's requirements for certain nutrients. Vitamins B_2, B_6, C and folic acid have so far been identified.[3]

63

Your baby's digestion

Digestion is the process of breaking down and transforming food so that it can be absorbed into the bloodstream for use in other parts of the body. With minor differences, the process is the same in babies as it is in adults. The diagrams below show the positioning of the principal organs involved, from the front and from the back.

The process starts in the mouth, where the salivary glands secrete the first digestive juices. The milk is then swallowed – by means of the muscular peristaltic motions of the esophagus – into the stomach, where gastric juices and muscular churnings continue its transformation. As a result, the solids in the milk – strands of protein and carbohydrate, globules of fat and microscopic vitamins and minerals – clump together to form curds. Being relatively solid, the curds remain for several hours in the stomach, where some of their nutrients are slowly absorbed into the blood. Meanwhile, the watery part of the milk, the whey, drains into the small intestine. In a young baby, the gastric juices usually contain all the enzymes needed to digest the nutrients in breast milk. The enzymes that are needed for digesting other foods only develop during the course of the first year of life. This is, of course, one reason why very early weaning is inadvisable.

Passing out of the stomach, the whey and, over the next hours, the curds, enter the small intestine, a long muscular tube that contracts rhythmically as the food moves along its path. Here, enteric (intestinal) juices and enzyme-rich bile from the liver break down the nutrients into even smaller molecules that are then absorbed into the intestinal wall. Blood vessels in the wall take up the absorbed nutrients which are carried to the liver for further processing, and to the lungs where oxygen is added. The heart then pumps the blood along the arteries, carrying the nutrients and oxygen to every cell in the body.

Whatever remains unabsorbed in the small intestine passes on to the large intestine (the *bowel* or *colon*), where it combines with other waste products of the body and is formed into stools by the bowel bacteria. In a young baby, the bowel empties under high pressure without any control. Only later is this developed.

Excretion of unused nutrients and other waste products also occurs in the urine, which is prepared in the kidneys. The two kidneys, situated just behind the stomach in the mid-back, filter blood as it circulates through the body, and regulate its composition. Whatever is not required in the blood is removed from it and passed out of the kidneys to the bladder. Urination in the young baby takes place frequently, and also without control. Very small quantities of other waste products are also excreted in the baby's breath, as well as through the skin.

The baby's excrement

During the first few days, a black, sticky substance, sometimes streaked with blood, is passed out of the baby's bowel. This is *meconium*, the baby's very earliest excrement, which contains the debris left over from what the baby swallowed in the womb.

After this come the first true stools, which are usually green, in a variety of shades. The reason for this is that the bowel, which was sterile at birth, is only gradually becoming populated with the bacteria needed to make normal stools. Breast milk contains tiny organisms that regulate this process and that soon start producing flocculent, yellowish, sweet-smelling stools, which turn slightly green in the air. Formulas cause rather different bacterial colonies, which produce quite firm, brown, foul-smelling stools, turning black in the air.

With urine, it is the concentration of the fluid which indicates whether all is well. In a healthy baby who has enough to drink, it will be dilute and therefore colorless and virtually odorless. The urine of a very young baby should flow copiously. If it does not, he may be dried out and in need of cooled, boiled water. If the weather is hot, or if he is developing a fever, the urine may be more concentrated and therefore yellow. It will stain the diaper and perhaps you will notice that it is causing a rash. If strong urine persists, consult a doctor because there may be an infection which requires medical treatment.

The position of the organs of your child's digestive system, from the front and the back.

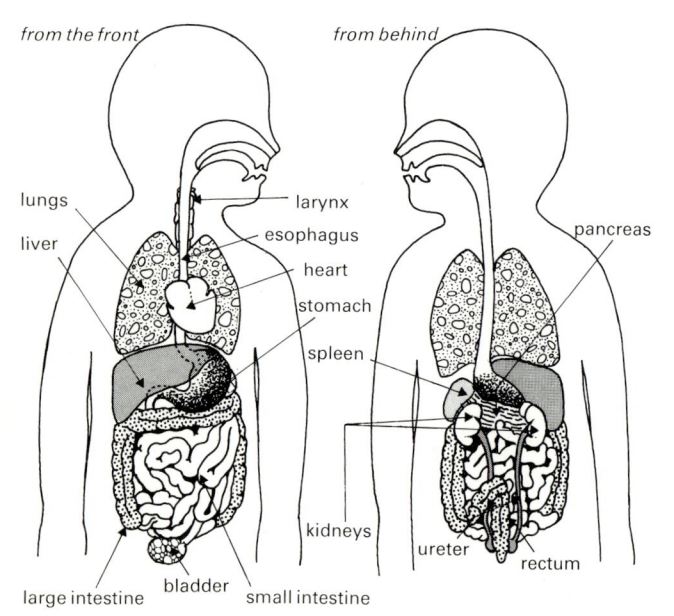

Burping and vomiting

Most babies swallow a certain amount of air with their milk, and sometimes this air gets trapped as bubbles within a mass of curds in the stomach. These bubbles may be released as a burp, either during the feeding or after it; but sometimes the bubbles build up and painfully stretch the stomach lining. If he starts fretting during or after a feed, put your baby on your shoulder halfway through the feeding and gently rub his lower back, perhaps patting a few times very gently. Burping or winding is a useful procedure, but if your feeding times are relatively calm, there may be no need for it.

If your baby drinks a little too much, he will bring up the surplus as a trickle of slightly curdled milk. If this happens regularly, your baby may perhaps be drinking too quickly. The calmer you are during his feedings, the less likely this is to happen.

Vomiting is something more vigorous. The curdled milk is thrown up into the baby's mouth and pours out. This may simply be the result of rough handling, because of over-enthusiastic burping, perhaps, or a diaper change before the food has settled in his stomach: but it may signify worse things. Periodic vomiting can occur in infection or if there is a lot of emotional tension in the air (babies are very sensitive to mood). It may also be due to the milk. If you are breastfeeding, check your own diet to see if you have eaten anything that might have upset the baby. If you are bottle-feeding and the vomiting recurs, you may need to change the formula.

Offer your baby periodic drinks of water on a teaspoon or from a bottle while you sort out what is happening. If the vomiting persists, and especially if the vomit is projected out of the baby's mouth, consult a doctor.

To minimize the risk of choking if your baby vomits in his sleep, place him on his stomach or his side. Very young babies who cannot turn over for themselves should never be put to sleep on their backs.

Coping with colic

During the first four months, your baby might start crying with great force and, despite his mother's best efforts to find out what is wrong, he may continue to cry and scream for several hours. His knees draw up to his chest, perhaps because of stomach cramps, perhaps simply as a part of his convulsive screaming. He seems to be in great pain. This is *colic*. A single outbreak can last up to six hours, and bouts tend to start at more or less the same time each day, often towards early evening.

It is doubtful that the baby is ill, for the outbreaks occur only at certain times of the day, and then only for a few hours. Nor is he hungry, for he has been offered the breast or the bottle and shows no interest. Nor is he thirsty, for he rejects the drink of water offered. His whole being is absorbed with one gigantic NO.

It is sometimes said that colic has no known cause and no effective treatment. This is not strictly true. Bottle-fed babies sometimes respond when they are put on a milk-free formula, which suggests that colic may be a symptom of cows' milk allergy. Breastfed babies, whose mothers have been drinking a lot of cows' milk, sometimes respond favorably when the mother removes milk from her diet.[1] A baby can inherit a cows' milk allergy from his mother, even though she may not know she is allergic, responding to the proteins in the cows' milk with painful intestinal cramps. Maternal allergies to tea, coffee, and chocolate are all also reported to be a cause of colic in some babies.

Emotional tension can also be the cause. We know one baby who had a colic attack every day when her father came home from work and her mother was hurrying to get his supper ready. Tension in the air? Another developed the symptoms just before nine each evening when her mother was getting ready to go to work. Protest? In both these cases, within days of the mothers realizing what was happening and changing the mood of that part of the day, the colic mysteriously disappeared.

But what do you do at the time? It can be terribly hard to stand that endless screaming without being able to help. Yet in the short term, there is little else to do. Your baby pushes you away, but at the same time he needs you there to prevent this chaotic experience from overwhelming him entirely. If you can, stay present but detached, periodically offering him the breast or a bottle of water. Try carrying him around in a baby-sling: this may rock him to sleep. From time to time, you may need someone else to stay with him so that you can take a break. Coping with colic requires a great deal of stamina.

In the longer run, try to solve the mystery. Observe the situation. When does the colic begin each day? What is *your* state of mind? What plans do you have for the next few hours? Who has just arrived or left? Keep a record and go through it at the end of the week. Babies are like emotional barometers: they know, in their bodies, when there is tension in the air. Some mothers do find a cause and can bring the colic to an end. Others report that the attacks disappear when the baby is about three or four months old. In a few cases, however, the colic continues through a good part of the first year.

Early feeding problems

Constipation

A baby who is feeding normally but only passes infrequent little pellets, and who cries with what could be the strain and pain of a blocked bowel, is constipated. This may have an emotional cause – some tension in the household, perhaps – and the possibility should be investigated before other actions are taken. Constipation can also have a physical cause and is relatively common among bottle-fed babies, perhaps as a result of the large quantities of iron used in many of the formulas.

Try easing the strain by offering plenty of cooled, boiled water to your baby. If bottle-feeding, you can try adding a little sugar to the bottle, which sometimes works in the short term. But avoid sugar as a regular addition to the formula. After a while, it will be ineffective against constipation, and at the same time it will give your baby a sweet tooth. A low-iron formula may also be effective but avoid changing more than once: simply changing the feed can itself cause constipation. From two months onwards, a little prune juice or diluted fruit juice may also be helpful. In addition, gentle but firm massage of the baby's abdomen along the course of his bowel can help soften any blockage. This involves a clockwise circular movement of your fingers around his abdomen or a counter-clockwise circular movement around his lower back. This will help press the stools on towards the anus.

If you think your baby is constipated, avoid getting into a spin about it. Some babies quite naturally let go of their stools only once or twice a week, building up to the great event with a day or so of excitement. Others let it all go thrice daily with ease. Before you start to do something, satisfy yourself that he really is in some distress. Your own anxiety, which the baby will sense, might only serve to constipate him more. If this becomes a problem for you, talk to other members of the family about it. Exchange views on constipation and see if your openness with each other has any effect on the baby's bowels. Perhaps tension is at the root of the matter.

Diarrhea

If your baby passes very frequent watery stools, he has diarrhea. In its mildest form, it passes in a day or two, a symptom of mild infection or some emotional upset. In breastfed babies, it may be caused by something the mother has eaten, in which case you should keep nursing, but check your diet. The diarrhea will probably pass as the milk returns to normal. In contrast, diarrhea caused by the formula is likely to persist because the formula remains constant in composition. The cream in cows' milk is often poorly digested, while the vegetable oils used instead of cream in the more modern formulas sometimes turn the stools very loose and green. You may need to try a different formula and, as long as the diarrhea persists, to offer extra bottles of cooled, boiled water to replace the water lost. Cooled peppermint or comfrey tea – traditional herbal remedies for diarrhea – can be offered to your baby from a spoon.

A small proportion of bottle-fed babies, between one and five percent, are allergic to the protein in cows' milk, which gives them diarrhea. Others cannot tolerate the milk lactose because of a rare disease called *galactosemia* in which the lactose-digesting enzyme, *galactose,* is lacking. The first signs of these conditions in young babies are vomiting after a feed or diarrhea. If the feeding is not then changed, there may be severe weight loss. These symptoms may be accompanied by skin rashes and difficulty in breathing.

A doctor will be able to arrange for the baby to be tested for allergy or intolerance, and to suggest an alternative formula if necessary. As about a third of the babies allergic to cows' milk are also allergic to soy milk, it may have to be a special product that is free of both. By the third month, a rice cereal or other milk-free weaning food can be introduced, and is usually well accepted.

As the best treatment of infantile cows' milk allergy or intolerance is a diet of breast milk, switch to breastfeeding if it is not too late. Some mothers manage this, in the same way as for breastfeeding an adopted baby, but it does take a lot of perseverance. Mothers of babies who have been ill from diarrhea and vomiting are sometimes too exhausted even to consider this possibility.

Babies with galactosemia are normally given a lactose-free formula, or one in which the lactose is predigested so that the digestive enzymes usually necessary are not required. Unlike cows' milk intolerance, which usually passes, with the baby often able to tolerate milk in his second or third year, galactosemia is, at present, a lifelong condition, and all milk products must therefore be eliminated from the diet.

Infantile gastroenteritis

If diarrhea continues for more than three or four days, the walls of the intestine, which are covered with tiny folds (the villi) to increase the surface area, become damaged and inflamed. The flow of enteric juices drops off and the amount of food that can be absorbed is reduced. This is *enteritis* or, because the stomach is usually involved, *gastroenteritis*. In the West, babies under six months of age are most commonly affected, sometimes as a result of infection, but more often from allergy or intolerance to the formula or as a result of it being too strong. In the Third World,

Early feeding problems

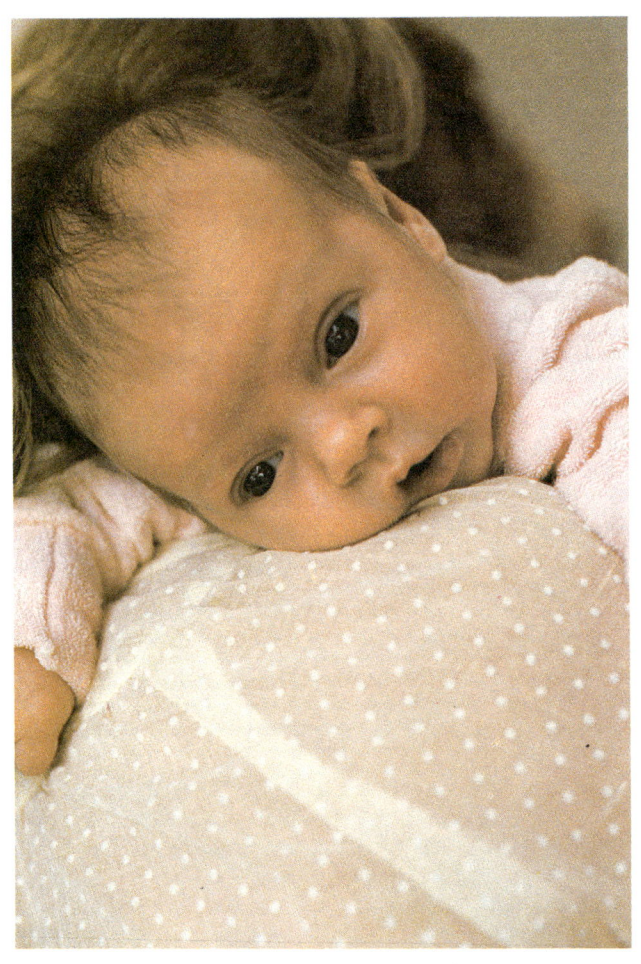

Babies are sensitive: make feeding as tranquil as you can.

where most young babies are breastfed, it is most common after weaning, when the child starts to drink contaminated water and to eat from the meager family pot. In those developing countries where the formulas are still widely used (the result of intensive formula sales tactics in the 1960s and 1970s), babies under six months are also at risk – not only because of allergy and incorrect mixing but also because the bottles tend to be made up with contaminated water. This can be fatal to a young baby. A major child health problem in the West, and the most widespread cause of childhood death in the Third World, gastroenteritis requires early treatment.[1] Always consult a doctor promptly.

The main risk is dehydration. The baby passes liquid stools many times a day, losing a lot of water and essential mineral salts in the process. Vomiting may increase this loss. He becomes very thirsty and – in his body's attempt to conserve fluids and minerals – his urine becomes sparse and concentrated. Gradually his body tissue dries out, and he appears shriveled, with sunken eyes and sunken fontanelles on top of the skull.

Dehydration can be prevented, and gastroenteritis can be treated, with rehydration salts. Dissolved in clean water, they can be given by mouth (oral salts) or, in an emergency, intravenously. Doctors in the West use salts made from a commercially prepared powder; but if these are not available, as frequently happens in the Third World, a mixture of sugar, salt and, if obtainable, baking soda and orange juice – all dissolved in cooled, boiled water – can be used.[2] This solution is given to the baby every few minutes, from a clean spoon or cup, until his urine is normal. Bottles should be used only if they are properly sterilized. If the baby vomits, you will need to wait for a few minutes before continuing. If the dehydration gets worse, or the baby does not urinate over a period of four hours, a doctor will be needed to give the solution intravenously. Rehydration salt solutions should ideally be used within twelve hours of being made up as bacterial growth increases after this period. They should always be kept in a cool, dark place and on no account be stored for more than twenty-four hours.[3]

REHYDRATION SALTS
(*dissolved in 1 liter of cooled, boiled water*)

COMMERCIAL MIXTURE
3.5 grams sodium chloride
2.5 grams sodium bicarbonate
1.5 grams potassium chloride
20 grams glucose

EMERGENCY HOMEMADE MIXTURE
¼ teaspoon common salt
¼ teaspoon baking soda
4 tablespoons orange juice
2 level tablespoons sugar

Rehydration salts are excellent first-aid. They can reduce the severity of diarrhea within hours, but frequently cannot cure the gastroenteritis. Infections can be treated with antibiotics, and faulty formula-mixing can be changed with education, but the problems of reinfection may be difficult to resolve. Clean drinking water is essential, as is sensible sanitation, with kitchen and toilet well separated.

When the diarrhea subsides, the baby should continue to be fed as much as possible. Breast milk is ideal, and it may not be too late for bottle-feeding mothers to switch to breastfeeding. If you continue with the bottle, the formula can be diluted if the baby vomits: use 1 part formula to 3 parts water (quarter-strength). When the vomiting has subsided, increase the strength to 2 parts of each (half-strength) for one day, and then start to feed with full-strength formula again.

Weight gain

At any time during his early months, your baby may start to grow very plump, with rolls of fat around his stomach, legs, and arms. This is usually nothing to worry about. Fat babies do not, as was widely thought during the 1970s, necessarily become fat children.[1,2] At that time, the theory was prevalent that overfed babies developed a larger than normal number of fat cells at a critical period of growth, and that this number is then fixed for life.[3] More recent studies have shown that critical periods for the development of fat cells can occur at any time in life, and that overfeeding in infancy tends to result in larger fat cells, which can at any time become smaller when the overfeeding stops. The chances of an overweight baby growing into a fat child are statistically about one in five.[4] But for that twenty percent, excess weight *is* a hazard to health and happiness. It predisposes the individual to diabetes and to heart disease, and also to endless teasing. Prevention is best.

Sometimes obesity is of genetic origin: a family trait that has little or nothing to do with the baby's diet.[1,2] If one of the parents is fat, there is an even chance that the baby will follow suit. If both parents are overweight, the odds are four to one that the baby will be, too. In other cases, obesity appears to result from overfeeding during pregnancy or, more commonly, from over-solicitous feeding during the early months.

Overfeeding

Over-solicitous feeding occurs when a baby does not really need food. This is unlikely to happen if you have come to know your baby relatively well and can distinguish his cries of hunger from cries of discomfort. But some mothers tend to offer a feeding whenever the baby cries, in the same way that they comfort themselves with a cup of tea or coffee, perhaps, when *they* are upset. Sometimes a mother will think her baby is hungry when she (the mother) is upset, and she does for the baby what she tends to do for herself in this situation: she feeds!

This kind of paradoxical scenario can be passed down through several generations before anyone notices. Yet perhaps the crying baby only wants a little company; or perhaps he is cold, or upset because someone else in the house is upset.

The effect of over-solicitous feeding appears to be different in breast and bottle-fed babies. When a breastfed baby sucks for comfort, the breast quickly reassures him and usually he will not take much milk. Indeed, if the last feeding was quite recent, there will not be much milk in the breasts as yet. So obesity in a breastfed baby is generally not due to overfeeding.

When a bottle-fed baby sucks for comfort, however, he simply receives more milk. If this happens frequently, he will tend to overfeed. Obese bottle-fed babies are sometimes starved of proper attention: the belly is full but the heart still hungers for 'nourishment'. If you are bottle-feeding and want to avoid this kind of situation, try non-food contact more often when your baby cries. Hold your baby, walk him around, play with him, rock him, sing to him; or simply lie down with him on your chest where he can hear the calming, familiar beat of your heart.

Overconcentrated feedings may also result in overfeeding. The mixing instructions on the package or the can have to be followed very carefully. Check that you add only the recommended amount of water, and not one more scoopful for good measure. Overconcentrated feedings may also give your baby diarrhea, and they will make him thirsty for water. If more milk is then given instead of water, a vicious overfeeding cycle will be set up.

A similar situation can occur if you add a spoonful of cereal to his bottle, perhaps because he seems unsatisfied with normal feedings, or perhaps because you think this will help him to sleep through the night. The feeding then becomes overconcentrated. With this practice, you also risk introducing your baby to foods that he may not yet be ready for. Many babies, for example, cannot digest wheat before the age of four months. There is no evidence that heavier meals make babies (or adults) sleep longer: and in general no solids should be introduced into the infant's diet until the fifth month.

If you think your baby may be obese, compare him with other babies you see in the street or at friends' houses, to put your impressions in perspective. You can also check his weight on a growth chart. If you are worried, consult your doctor or pediatrician.

To some extent, you can slow down the growth of a bottle-fed baby by offering him water when you feel he has taken what he needs, especially in summer when he may be thirstier than usual. If he wants more milk afterwards, you can always go back to the formula.

Underfeeding

In our society, underfeeding is rare; and when it does occur, it is usually a result of the baby losing his appetite because of illness. Recovery from the illness is normally accompanied by a return of appetite. But it can also happen that a breastfeeding mother's milk supply declines, as a result of her own tiredness; and without her realizing it at first, the baby may be consequently under-fed. If you are finding breastfeeding, and life in general, a strain, and your baby seems

Weight gain

unsatisfied, it could be that your milk supply has been reduced to below what he needs. If you want to continue feeding, complete rest and a well-balanced diet are required. Give your relationship with the baby priority and delegate as many of your chores to others as you can. Let him suck whenever he wants to. This will help increase your milk supply.

You may be advised to introduce night feedings of formula, both to give the baby extra food and to give you the chance to rest. But if you do this, your milk supply is unlikely to increase. On the contrary: lacking that additional sucking stimulus, the milk supply will probably decrease. In addition, the introduction of formula to the baby's digestive system may make him less able to absorb some of the nutrients in breast milk. Introduce bottles only if you are ready to start the weaning process.

Bottle-fed babies can be underfed, too. Apart from overdilution of the formula, the holes in the nipples may be too small, so that the baby simply cannot get enough milk. The holes must be big enough so that a steady stream of bubbles rises in the bottle as the baby drinks. If you fear that your baby is underweight, check his progress on the growth chart or ask your doctor about it.

Weighing in

Weighing your baby once a week will certainly give some idea of his rate of physical growth, but it says relatively little of his health and emotional development. The quality of his skin, his alertness and the sparkle in his eyes will give you a better indication of his progress. Nevertheless, by plotting your baby's weight each month against the average range on a standard growth chart, you will have regular reassurance that all is well: while if his weight curve starts to move out of the average range, it will alert you and your doctor to the possibility that all is not well.

During the first week after birth, breastfed babies drink very little and usually lose a pound or so. In contrast, bottle-fed babies (and especially those who are fed full-strength formula from the start) usually gain weight straight away. They also normally grow more rapidly than breastfed babies throughout the first year. Some bottle-feeding mothers welcome this, as if it were an advantage. It can, after all, be tempting to want your baby to gain weight at least as fast as (and maybe faster than) other women's babies. The trouble with this kind of competition is that a baby becomes prized because of his size. Everybody has his or her own internal biological growth program. If you feed your baby according to his hunger and let him grow at his individual speed, he is far more likely to be healthy and happy.

Plotting your baby's curve on the chart provides a record of progress. Each infant grows at his own pace, but his curve should be more-or-less parallel with the average curve and within the average weight range.

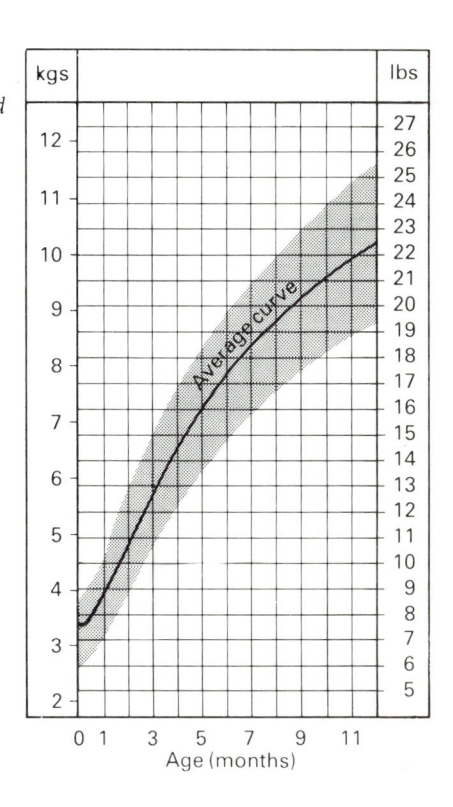

Ideally, his weight will start and remain within the average range on the chart: and although the curve will probably not be absolutely smooth, it should run more or less parallel to the average. If he was born very heavy or very light, his curve should grow towards the average curve.

Low-birth-weight (LBW) babies tend to drink more and grow faster than average, so that by the second year they have largely caught up and are within the average range. Conversely, very heavy newborn babies sometimes grow more slowly than average during the first six months, until they are within the average range.

When a baby's growth curve starts to rise up out of the average range, he is probably putting on too much weight and may well be overeating. On the other hand, if the curve flattens off, he is probably underfeeding and may be ill. As soon as his milk intake goes up, because his health has recovered or other problems have been rectified, the curve will rise steeply to its original path.

A growth chart is simple to use. Your baby's age is plotted along the horizontal axis; weight is plotted vertically. Each month, his weight can then be marked by a cross above the appropriate age: the crosses are joined together so that a growth curve is gradually built up. The curve on the chart shows an ideal rate of progress, although in reality half of all babies will have a curve above it and half below. However, ninety percent of all babies will have curves that fall within the average range, as shaded. An example is provided for use on page 89.

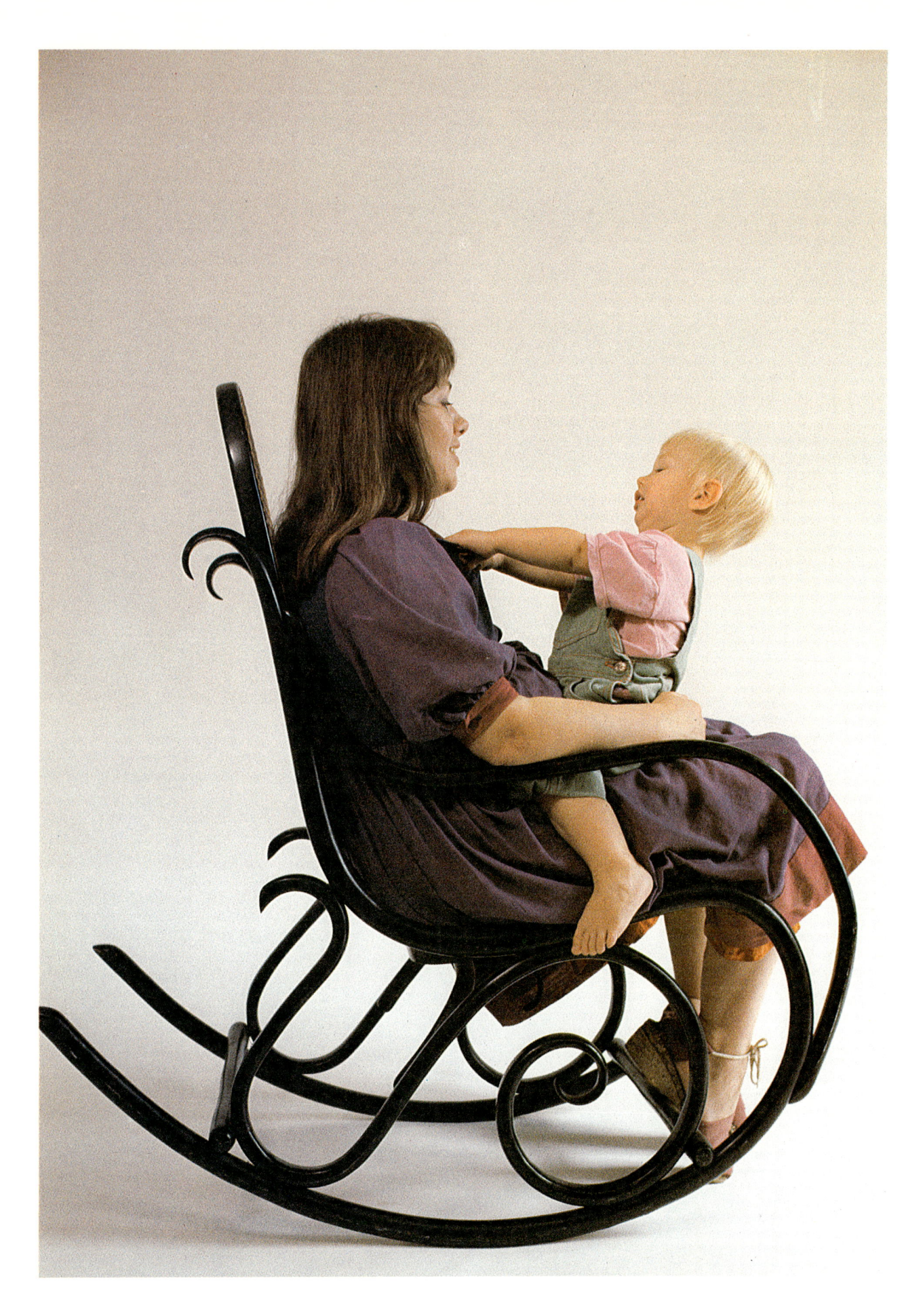

PART 3

The weaning process

Ideally, weaning should be a natural process: something that develops *between* you and your baby, not something you *do* to him. Or course, you may have to help the process along, just as you help him adapt to everything else in this strange, new world into which he has been born: but there is no need to rush the process. Weaning tends only to happen easily when the baby is physically and emotionally ready for it.

Based on the old English word *wenian*, meaning 'to accustom', weaning involves a separation of mother from baby. The French word for weaning, *sevrage*, actually means 'separation'. The process involves the baby in learning to cope with the world beyond his mother and in adapting to the customs of that world. Food plays a vital part in this process. But dietary change is only part of the story.

Your baby, given all the milk he needs, will probably be ready to taste new foods at between four and six months, and to do without the breast or bottle as his principal nourishment by the end of his first year. Earlier weaning is inadvisable. It forces the issue, and can often leave a baby frustrated and insecure. Premature weaning – before your baby is physically and mentally ready for it – may cause problems for both of you.

Growth and development

While the newborn baby lives in a sort of dream world, without making distinctions and without a sense of himself as a separate person, he has by about four months begun to awaken to what we adults call 'reality'. Different objects become clearly distinguishable, and so do people. Although he has been familiar with your voice and heartbeat since long before birth, he now begins to see you as a person in your own right. This can be immensely exciting for both of you. He starts to look at you with a different kind of interest and begins to communicate with you in his own infantile way.[1]

At this stage, breastfed babies start to transfer their amorous attentions from the breast to the mother as a whole, and bottle-fed babies from the bottle to whoever is holding it. If you usually attend to feeding yourself, a new depth will grow between you and the baby. For he is now beginning to understand in a conscious way that you are his 'home base', as indeed you have been from the moment he was conceived. The recognition of a home base is vitally important to his sense of security. It forms the basis of all his early journeys in life, once he learns to crawl and to walk. Babies who have been given bottles by a number of people tend to lack this important home base feeling.

Physical development matches these emotional and mental developments. Your baby rapidly acquires a wide range of movements that give him greater mobility and flexibility. He learns to stretch his limbs at will, to direct them and coordinate them. He learns to grasp things in a purposeful way, and most of what he grasps – by careful coordination of his muscles and eyes – he begins to carry to his mouth. For his mouth is his great 'explorer'. It is not that he wants to *eat* his wooden rattle or his furry bunny: he simply needs to explore them with his highly sensitive tongue, lips, gums, and palate.

Standing up for himself

By the end of their first year, many babies are able to crawl with speed about the home. They explore every accessible place, reaching as far and as high as they can. Everything and everyone seems to interest them. They learn to stand: a milestone not only for you as a proud parent but also for the baby in his own right. Of course, he is still highly dependent on you and will be for many years to come: but now he can explore further afield and can probably cope for short periods without you, not asleep, but confidently facing the world on his own. The development of this self-confidence will be of the greatest possible importance to him in life. In contrast, an insecure child explores with trepidation, tends to be afraid of strangers and cannot easily cope with his mother's absences. Without the restoration of trust and confidence, insecure babies grow into insecure adults, still feeling, albeit unconsciously, that the center of their world is not 'self' but 'mother'.

Letting go

In many Third World communities, you can observe the natural process of weaning. All you need is time, for the gradual transition from the breast to solids is allowed to take place over several years. Nutritionist A.K. Rahman and sociologist Barbara Thompson, in their classic study of weaning among African mothers in Gambia, reported that all newborn babies receive the breast as their main food, with other easily digested foods being introduced during the first year. At between four and five months, a watery rice gruel and seasonal fruit are offered. By seven or eight months, fresh grains (boiled rice or steamed millet) replace the gruel: and by the end of the first year, either a peanut sauce is given with the grains, or fish, or goats' milk. Breast milk continues to be the major source of nutrients into the second year, when it is gradually replaced by increased amounts of cooked food and raw fruit.[2]

Most of these babies continue to have breast milk into the third year, when they either relinquish the breast voluntarily, or the milk dries up. Alternatively, the mothers leave their toddlers with a relative in a neighboring village for several days. Only when these forcibly separated babies are able to play with the mother without going for her breasts are they considered weaned and taken home again. Some mothers prefer not to be separated from their toddlers, but mock them for as long as they continue to want the breast. Some even paint their nipples with pepper or mud, in an attempt to turn the baby's interest away. Sometimes a mother has to be cruel to be kind.

Premature weaning

In recent years, most babies in the modern world have been introduced to weaning cereals and other foods during their first three or four months, and were entirely weaned by six months.[3] This was due partly to a change in fashion and partly to the lifestyle of modern mothers, who were more likely to want to wean early, perhaps because there was a job to return to, or because child-rearing in isolation, without the support of a close-knit group of women friends and relatives, was a lonely and exhausting experience. Yet the situation has not always been like this. At the turn of the century, most mothers still breastfed their babies for a year or more. By the 1930s, the recommended age for weaning was six to eight months. By the 1940s, it was four to six months; and by the 1950s, weaning within the first month was considered quite proper. Only with the discovery, in the late 1960s and early 1970s, that unmodified cows' milk, wheat, eggs, and certain other foods can make a very young baby ill, was the recommended age raised. Now, four to six months is once again widely accepted by most medical authorities as the minimum age at which to set weaning in motion.

Premature weaning is associated with certain physical risks. Allergy to cows' milk, wheat, corn, berries, fish, egg white, and orange juice have all been reported.[4] And for the breastfed baby, the early introduction of other foods, including formula, will also change the digestive pattern of whatever breast milk remains in the diet. For example, the introduction of iron-rich foods, or manufactured foods enriched with iron, immediately decreases the baby's capacity to absorb iron from breast milk.[5] In addition, the natural antibacterial effect of breast milk iron is reduced as soon as the bowel is swamped with other forms of iron.[5]

The emotional risks of premature weaning are less well documented than the physical risks, though they appear to resemble the effects of formula-feeding by the clock. The baby's natural sense of appetite is taken over by the mother, who decides both *what* he shall eat and *when*. Professor Hilde Bruch of Texas University has pointed out in her psychiatric case studies of obese adults that this loss of self-regulation in early childhood can be a fundamental cause of obesity.[6]

Many babies can tolerate a selected range of foods by six months. But if you and the baby are well and happy with your milk feedings, you should not feel under pressure to introduce new foods until later in the first year. Once you start to do so, the process of weaning will be irreversibly underway. This means that the more your breastfed baby eats of other foods, the less your milk supply will be. If your milk supply does seem to be drying up and you still want to continue breastfeeding, you will need complete rest and a very good diet, according to the maxim 'Feed the Mother, and thereby the Child'.

A mother at home with a small baby, and perhaps with other children, leads a demanding and sometimes very lonely existence. In this respect, she is different from mothers in a pre-industrial society, where the generations would live together and a breastfeeding mother would have all the support and guidance of the family and the community. If you find your life turning into a succession of broken nights and haunted days – which sends millions of mothers to the doctor during the first year after a birth – you may feel like weaning speedily. If this is the case, get all the help you can from a breastfeeding counselor, from the La Leche League or a similar organization, or from another breastfeeding mother. It might provide just the encouragement you need to keep going for a month or two longer.

If you have to return to work very soon, however, premature weaning may be unavoidable for you. Some mothers continue to provide their milk, expressing it at home and at work, to be fed to the baby while they are away: but most opt for early weaning on to a formula.

If you have to wean your baby during the first four months, give yourself as much time for the transition as possible. Most babies do not like sudden change. If you cannot avoid weaning in a very short period of time, try to be with your baby as often as possible. This will reassure him that, although his familiar breast or bottle has gone, his mother has not.

Weaning from the bottle

Bottle-fed babies are very commonly taking other foods by their fourth month. The transition from formula to weaning cereals does not involve such a spectacular change in their diet. Indeed, it may only involve adding another powder (the cereal) to the powder you already feed the baby (the formula), and offering spoonfuls instead of drinks. But do avoid putting cereals into the bottle. Your baby needs to learn how to eat, not to be tricked into drinking an extra-rich food.

Many mothers believe that a bottle-fed baby should be allowed to keep the bottle as long as he wants to do so: but the introduction of new foods provides a good opportunity to wean him slowly off it. Once the first year is over, a baby who still gets a bottle may cling to it for the next four or five years. If you cannot avoid an endless succession of bottles, at least avoid putting soft drinks in them or your baby's mouth will be continually bathed in tooth-rotting sugary fluids. Even fruit juice can cause dental plaque.

Another pregnancy

A healthy, well-nourished breastfeeding mother can continue to suckle one child, while nourishing another infant in her womb. In some societies, there is a taboo against this: but if you find yourself pregnant while your first baby is still very young, you need not feel bound to accelerate weaning. Some mothers enjoy breastfeeding while they are pregnant and find it relaxing. Others complain that they are overtired or that their nipples are too sore to continue.

A flexible weaning program

Our weaning program follows four principal phases, and the foods we recommend are basically whole, unrefined, and unprocessed. If you can introduce your baby to these right from the start, they will give him a balanced diet as the breast or the bottle gradually disappears from his life.

THE FOUR PHASES OF WEANING

1. Introducing new tastes
2. Introducing new meals
3. Replacing the breast or bottle
4. Phasing out the breast or bottle

When to start

If you follow our program, you will be feeding your baby nothing but breast milk or formula for the first four to six months, but will begin to offer him a taste of other foods towards the end of that period. By the seventh month, you may be preparing him one meal a day, including some of these new foods. By nine months, two meals may replace his milk: and by the end of the first year, most of his nourishment will probably be coming from other foods. The timing of the final disappearance of breast milk from his diet will probably depend on you, although some babies do seem to lose interest quite spontaneously. If you have let the weaning process develop naturally, instead of bringing it forward, this may not occur until the second year. In general, the flow of breast milk declines as other foods take its place in the baby's diet and his sucking decreases. With bottle-feeding, the point at which you call a stop will depend not on the supply of formula, which is unlimited, but more simply on how you, your baby, and perhaps his father feel about it.

Remember that physical and mental development follow their own particular timing in each baby. One baby may have ten teeth at his first birthday, while another has not even a bump on his gums. One baby grows quickly at first and then slows down, while another has a growth spurt late in the first year. One is naturally confident and this confidence has been nurtured so that he takes easily to new foods; another seems to be anxious, perhaps because he was not given all the support he needed during the early months, so that now he is reluctant to try new foods. Each baby must embark on the bridge between infancy and childhood at his own pace. Follow your baby's signals as much as you can. The closer you are to him, the easier it will be for him, and for you, to make the crossing.

PHASE ONE   Introducing new tastes
(four to seven months)

As your baby nears the end of this first half-year, he will probably start showing an interest in new foods. If you offer him a scraping of mashed banana, avocado or peach, or a slice of apple or pear, he is likely to try it with interest. Raw, natural foods, intended not as meals but simply as something to taste, are an ideal introduction to the delights of real food: and if he enjoys them, he will soon be back for more.

Next, you will probably want to see how he reacts to cooked food. Perhaps you sometimes sit down to meals with him in your lap, and he seems to be interested in what you are eating. He wants to know what that stuff is that you devour with such pleasure! All you need to do is pick a meal where the foods are simple and bland. It might be a dish of boiled carrots, potatoes or rice, or perhaps some stewed apple. Mash up a little, and offer it to him. Leave out the salt or any other flavorings you might want for yourself. His taste buds are incredibly sensitive; you can get an idea what he could be tasting if you fast for a day and then eat a boiled carrot or, better still, a peach. The flavor, you will find, is extraordinarily clear. You can gradually introduce him to the stronger tastes of seasoning, as he grows.

Manufactured weaning foods

Manufactured weaning foods are all too often a sad introduction to the wonderful world of food that lies beyond the breast or bottle. Like the formulas, many consist simply of powder or flakes that become a meal when you add liquid. They often contain added nutrients like iron and calcium, although nothing like the range of vitamins and minerals added to formula or naturally present in fresh, unrefined foods. The ingredients are normally medically approved, so from a biochemical point of view they are adequate, and they are always manufactured in conditions of the utmost hygiene. But the taste and textures tend to be dull and lifeless, and quite unlikely to stimulate your baby to any great enthusiasm for 'real' food. If your family diet contains a lot of refined foods, you may tend to choose boxes and jars of babyfood during the next few months, but try to include a few fresh foods.

Meanwhile, be wary of teething biscuits. There are two kinds: those like brittle toast (Zwieback), usually made of flour and water, which serve quite well as something edible for the baby to gnaw on with his gums or first teeth; and those like sweet crisp biscuits that can either be eaten dry or dissolved in milk to form a porridge. The latter may contain up to one third sugar, which is the last thing your baby should be eating.

A flexible weaning program

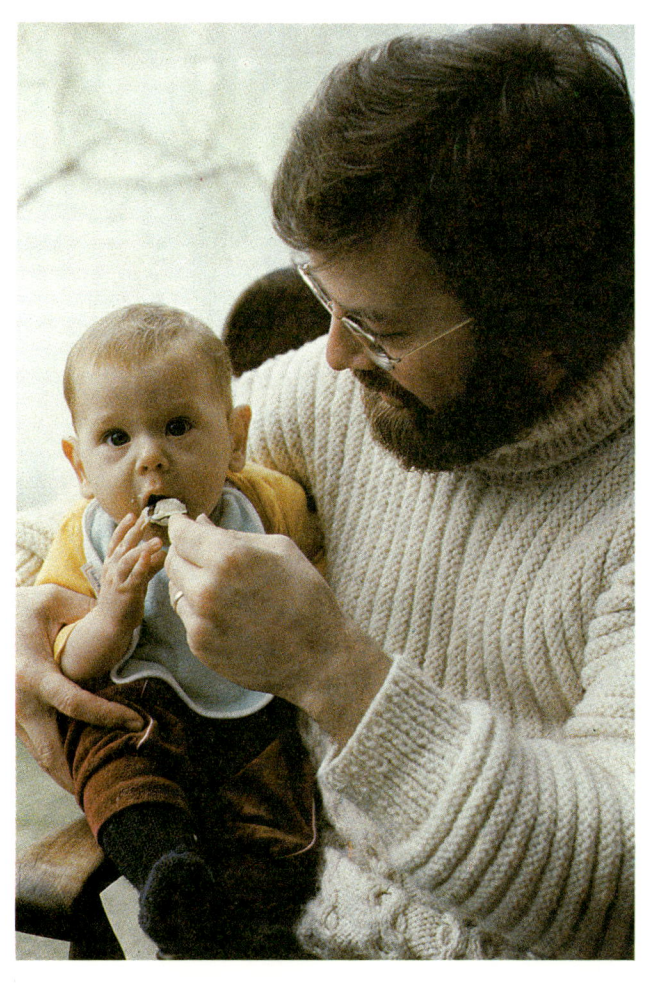

Weaning begins, and with it all the excitement of new tastes.

PHASE TWO   Introducing new meals
(*six to nine months*)

Once your baby is happily accepting bits of new food, you can start to offer him larger quantities. This is the beginning of his gradual transition from the breast or bottle to solid food. For the breastfeeding mother, it also starts the gradual decrease in milk supply. As your baby will normally be hungry at the start of a feeding, let him have the breast or bottle first. Then, when he takes a break, offer some other food on a small spoon or on your finger. If he is interested, the rest of his meal may well come from the spoon, although he may want to finish up with the bottle or at the breast again.

A finely ground-up purée is best at this stage: semi-solids that he half-drinks, half-eats. You can use any of the foods he has accepted so far, either singly or in combination. A small electric blender or manual food mill is virtually essential: lumps tend to cause indigestion or vomiting before chewing is mastered. Mixtures of boiled rice and steamed vegetables, or fruit and yogurt are excellent starters. These two types of dish – one savory, one sweet – have a hundred different variations depending upon which vegetables or fruit you use. Mashed potato with butter or margarine, scrambled eggs, and low-salt cottage cheese are also usually accepted at this stage. If you are offering egg, milk or yogurt for the first time, keep an eye open for allergic reactions. These foods can cause rashes, indigestion, or breathing difficulties in susceptible babies. Ground-up chicken or ocean fish are also suitable. Red meats are rather heavy and fibrous, though their broth is usually easy to digest.

At this phase of weaning, your baby still gets most of his nourishment from the breast or his formula, so you do not need to worry about his new diet being balanced. At the same time, introduce him to the kind of foods that you would like him to be eating later on. And remember, when food is scarce, as it is at times for the lowest income families, your baby can be adequately fed on a mixture of whole grains and legumes, with small quantities of dark green leafy vegetables, fruit, and occasional animal foods. Below are recipes for two basic types of first meal.

Rice and vegetable purée with cheese

1 cup rice, preferably brown, well-cooked
1 cup mixed vegetables, steamed or boiled
½ cup vegetable broth, milk, or water
1 raw egg yolk (optional)
1 teaspoon sunflower margarine or butter (optional)
1 teaspoon grated cheese

1. Warm rice and vegetables in the broth, milk, or water.
2. Stir in the egg yolk for a richer mixture.
3. Purée the warm mixture in a blender or hand-grinder.
4. For older babies, grind the purée less finely and add a few vegetable chunks.
5. Stir in margarine or butter, if used.
6. Serve topped with grated cheese.

Fruit and yogurt purée

½ cup fresh soft fruit, mashed (not berries)
or cooled, stewed hard fruit, such as apples
or soaked dried fruit such as apricots or prunes, with stones removed
2 tablespoons unsweetened yogurt, plain
1 tablespoon cream (optional)

1. Prepare fruit by mashing, soaking, or cooking.
2. Purée fruit (with some cooking or soaking in water if necessary).
3. Stir in yogurt and, for a richer mixture, add cream.

A flexible weaning program

PHASE THREE Replacing breast or bottle
(eight to twelve months)

As the weaning progresses, your baby will gradually be eating two and then three meals a day. The speed at which this happens will depend very much on you *and* the baby. The more new foods he eats, the less breast or bottle milk he will be getting; and – if things are to go smoothly – this needs to be what both of you want. If you try to hurry the process along, he may start refusing what only a few days ago he was happy to accept. When you sit down to a meal together, take your cues from him about how often to give him a spoonful or when to give him a drink of water. If you can stand the mess, let him have the spoon so that he can start to try feeding himself. He may not get much into his mouth at first, but practice will help.

Bottle-feeding babies often reach this stage more quickly than breastfed babies, perhaps because they are already accustomed to foods that do not come from the mother's body. There is indeed a case for saying that bottle-fed babies are weaned as soon as they learn to do without the breast. They also tend to learn more quickly that the night is not a good time for them to eat, and they adapt by taking a slightly larger evening feeding before they sleep, to last them through the night. Breastfed babies, even when they are eating two or three meals a day, usually tend to wake more often at night until the second year.

As new foods gradually provide a larger proportion of your baby's diet, it becomes important that the new diet is properly balanced. You can no longer rely on his first food to supply all that he needs. Using your own balanced diet as a guide, set out to give him three well-balanced dishes each day. The savory purée that served him well in Phase Two can continue as one meal, enriched with extra oil or butter and animal foods or legumes as time goes by. A second meal could be a sugar-free weaning granola, which is an excellent staple food for small children; and a third could be something from one of your own daily meals, perhaps slightly modified at first.

A weaning granola is made of rolled (and thus partly cooked) grains, like oats and wheat, nuts dried fruit and seeds, with stewed or mashed fresh fruit for variety and extra vitamins. Cooked with milk or water, it makes an excellent staple dish which can partly replace the breast or bottle.

The family meals you share with your baby will need to be relatively simple ones at first: scrambled or boiled eggs, baked potatoes with cheese, chicken or fish, or a thick vegetable soup. If necessary, simply grind up a portion for him before adding salt, spices, or sauces for yourself. You can then gradually experiment by offering him spicier dishes if that is the way you normally eat. (You can be sure he will spit it out if it is too strong). As he learns to chew, you can leave chunks of vegetables, egg, and fish in his bowl. But make sure they are cut quite small at first.

Desserts need not be an everyday affair. To your baby, a sweet dish can constitute a whole meal. A purée of cooked fruit can be enriched with milk or yogurt; finely grated raw apple or mashed banana can be mixed into a little left-over granola or served alone with a teaspoon of orange or lemon juice for extra Vitamin C. There is no need for extra sugar!

By the end of Phase Three, your baby will be getting most of his food from new dishes and relatively little from the breast or bottle. You may be giving him his old fundamental food only once or twice each day, perhaps early in the morning and in the evening to help him on his way to sleep. If you have been breastfeeding, you do not need to introduce a bottle. Many babies accept a drinking cup straight away.

Weaning granola (a staple dish)

4 tablespoons rolled oats/wheat
1 tablespoon mixed nuts/sunflower seeds
1 tablespoon raisins or sultanas
1 cup milk or milk-and-water

1. Grind dry ingredients to a coarse powder in a blender.
2. Transfer powder to a saucepan, and add the liquid.
3. Stirring constantly, bring the mixture to a boil.
4. Reduce the heat and simmer for 2–4 minutes until smooth.

For variation:

1. Stir in mashed banana or finely grated apple before serving: or
2. Add a few drops of lemon juice for flavor and for Vitamin C: or
3. Add egg yolk or a pat of butter to encourage weight gain.

Steamed white fish (*use a bamboo steaming tray or a sieve*)

Small fillet of fresh, flat white fish
½ teaspoon butter or margarine
A few drops lemon juice (optional)

1. Heat a little water in a small saucepan.
2. Place the fish skin-down in a steaming tray or sieve.
3. Place the steaming tray or sieve over the saucepan so that the fish is above the water.
4. Cover with a lid and steam for 5–7 minutes.
5. Remove the fish from the steaming tray.
6. Skin the fish, add butter or margarine and, if you like, lemon juice.

Tooth development will be one indication of the foods your baby will welcome. With the eruption of the first milk teeth, he is preparing to bite. Offer chunks of cooked vegetables, peeled cucumbers, hard cheese, and fruit. If you make him granola, grind it less finely, and give him peeled soft fruits. When his back, chewing teeth come through – probably not until his second year – he will be able to cope with pieces of meat, harder fruits, partly-cooked vegetables and bread. You can keep his teeth free from food scraps, which might turn bad, by always giving him a drink after the meal and brushing his teeth.

PHASE FOUR   Phasing out the breast or bottle
(nine months onwards)

Breastfed babies sometimes lose interest in the breast during their first year; others want to keep sucking well into the second year, even though their diet now contains plenty of other foods. There is give and take in any relationship, and there will be a time when either you or he will have had enough, perhaps both of you together. You do not have to paint your nipples with pepper like the Gambian women. If your baby does not like the idea of parting with the breast, you can simply say 'no' and stick to your decision.

If you have been bottle-feeding, you probably substituted ordinary milk for the formula about halfway through the first year, and may have weaned your baby off his bottle at the same time or soon afterwards, perhaps by giving him a new cup instead. If you did not, the chances are that he will now be extremely attached to the bottle, and it may be hard to get him to give it up. If this has happened, try not to force him. You can avoid having half-empty bottles of souring milk about the house by giving him only water or diluted juices in the bottle and insisting that he take milk – if you give him milk – from a cup. Remember not to put full-strength fruit juices or anything containing sugar in the bottle, since this provides an ideal solution for the growth of bacteria on his teeth.

If your own diet is well-balanced, and you are providing the same sort of foods for your baby, his diet will also be balanced. You do not need to pump him with protein, as was widely recommended during the 1950s and 1960s, both for babies and for beef cattle; but every meal should contain some complete protein: milk, cheese, or yogurt; egg, fish, poultry, or meat; or a mixture of grains and legumes.

Whole, fresh cows' and goats' milk are normally well tolerated by a six-month-old baby: but the more that he drinks, the greater the risk of allergic reaction. Professor Herbert Barrie of the Charing Cross Hospital, London, has calculated that five eight-ounce bottles or two-and-a-half U.S. pints of milk a day (which is what some babies are drinking by this time) is the equivalent on a weight-for-weight basis of an adult drinking twenty pints of milk a day. "This is a sure prescription for wheezy bronchitis, vomiting, and rashes", he concludes. In addition, some babies develop intestinal bleeding as a result of drinking a lot of milk, with subsequent diarrhea and loss of nutrients.

Moderate amounts of milk (two or three cups per day) will supply your baby with a range of nutrients, especially protein and calcium. But because cows' milk naturally contains little of Vitamins A, C, and D, and little iron, his diet should contain other natural food sources of these nutrients, or supplements. In the United States, cows' milk is fortified with Vitamins A and D.

Nutrients present at very low levels in unmodified milk and where else to find them

Iron: meat, especially liver and kidneys; shellfish and eggs; whole grains, especially bran and wheat germ; dark green leaves of chard, spinach, kale, watercress; legumes, especially kidney, lima and soybeans, lentils, peanut and sesame butter (tahina); gooseberries and apricots; dried fruit

A daily helping of at least two iron-rich foods is advisable.

Vitamin C: oranges, lemons, plums, papaya, avocado, potatoes

A daily wedge of orange to chew on is sufficient.

Vitamin A: liver (meat or fish), cod-liver oil; dark green leaves of spinach, turnips; full-fat dairy produce, especially butter, fatty cheese; carrots, sweet potatoes, peaches, and apricots; fortified margarine or milk, eggs

A daily portion of two of these is recommended

Vitamin D: fish, especially herring, mackerel, sardines, tuna, salmon; fish liver, and cod-liver oil; fortified margarine, egg yolk;

A new balance

Towards the end of the weaning process, your baby will be getting most of his nourishment from new foods. Occasionally, he may still need the reassurance of your breast or a bottle of his old familiar formula: but, by and large, he can probably manage very well without them now.[1]

If you have been able to balance your own diet, and you offer your toddler only the kinds of food you eat, his intuitive senses of hunger and appetite will tell you what he needs. The classic experiments of Dr. Clara Davis in the 1930s showed this clearly. She worked with a group of orphans between six months and four years of age, offering them free choice from a wide range of a natural, unprocessed foods. Milk, buttermilk, boiled eggs, a variety of cooked grains, raw and cooked vegetables, meats and fish dishes were all available. No food was salted, but salt was available separately. At first, the children ate in what appeared to be quite a haphazard manner. One child ate eleven eggs in a day, another ate thirteen bananas. But over a period of several weeks, all had selected a balanced diet for themselves. Dr. Davis commented that "the trick, if trick you wish to call it, was in the food list. Confined to natural, unprocessed foods as it was, and without any made dishes of any sort, it reproduced the conditions under which primitive peoples intuitively select a scientifically sound diet".[2]

In our experience, toddlers who become used to highly processed foods, and especially to high salt and sugar intake, do not have this intuitive power to select what they need. Their appetites have been spoiled. This does not mean that you have to screen your child from the world of sugary foods and potato chips: but you can do him (and yourself) a favor by keeping them to a minimum.

Meanwhile, give him the breast or a bottle of formula when he seems to need it. All babies, and not a few adults, regress from time to time, returning to the mentality of an earlier period and wanting more 'babyish' foods. If you can go along with this, your toddler will not need to become frantic or withdraw into some form of illness to get what he needs.

Snacks and meals

If you observe regular mealtimes, then you will probably have taught your baby to expect the same: whereas if your own habits are more flexible, the baby may have followed you or simply established an appetite schedule of his own. There is no right or wrong in this. Nor is there any particular nutritional advantage in the toddler only eating at mealtimes, unless this is the only occasion when nourishing food is available to him, or unless you have no opportunity to offer him food at other times.

Be as flexible as you can. You do not need to slave all day in the kitchen to be a good mother. Although cooking is an ancient act of mothering, and an important one, the frustration and resentment of having to prepare an endless succession of meals can poison your life and, in a sense, the food itself. If you find yourself constantly in the kitchen, you may also start to overeat. So take it easy! Your baby can be just as well-nourished if you replace one meal each day with a snack.

Suitable snacks during the second year include cubes of bread and butter, hard cheese, hard fruits, slices of cucumber and tomato, soft fruits, and cottage cheese. They should be easy to handle. The more your toddler can exercise his growing jaw and teeth, the healthier they will be.

Snacks are also good when you are out and about, but watch out! Take-out foods from fast-food restaurants, bakeries, hot-dog stands, and ice cream trucks are often indigestible for young children. They also tend to be made with the kind of ingredients you would never buy: cheap saturated cooking fats, starchy fillers, and additives. And they often contain large quantities of sugar.

So when you go out with your baby, be prepared: take a container of yogurt and a banana with you, or a wholewheat roll, an apple, and a piece of cheese: you can always find a spot for a stroller meal. As the third year approaches, you can add occasional ice creams, potato chips, and hot-dogs, the sort of foods he will see other children eating in the street and will almost certainly want to try: but avoid them for as long as possible. If you totally deny him these refined foods, he may become obsessed with them.

Sugary foods

Eaten in quantity, sugar becomes addictive. Toddlers who are used to snacking on sugary foods may please their mothers by eating well and putting on weight, but they are also developing the kind of eating habits that lead to malnutrition in later life. As we have seen, high sugar consumption is one of the hallmarks of a society that suffers from a number of degenerative diseases – including atherosclerosis and diabetes, as well as dental decay – and excessive sugar intake is thought to be one of the prime causes of such conditions.[1,2]

The most widespread of the sugar diseases is undoubtedly dental decay. In the West, we consume an average of two pounds of sugar a week each, about as much as our grandparents ate in a year. The state of our teeth is equally startling. By the age of five, three-quarters of all

British children suffer from dental problems, with an average of five decayed, missing, or filled teeth. This average doubles for children in their late teens and trebles by their late twenties. By the age of fifty, half the people in Britain have lost all their teeth. Sugar is certainly not the only cause but it is, equally certainly, an important one.

In the United States, the pattern is similar. Only ten percent of two-year-olds suffer from dental caries, but by the end of the fourth year this has risen to a startling fifty-seven percent.[3] This fairly sudden rise in caries during the third year of life reflects both dietary changes and the fact that it takes about two years for newly erupted teeth to turn bad. It may be some consolation that the first teeth will be replaced by permanent ones, but after that there are no more.

The process of dental decay is interesting. Teeth have two main components: a relatively soft, living matrix and the hard, mineralized 'cement' that fills the matrix. Around the borderline of the teeth and gums there collects a mixture of worn-out gum cells, normal mouth bacteria, and food debris. This is *plaque*. In itself, plaque is harmless: but when the teeth are exposed to sugar for any length of time, the bacteria convert the sugar into acids that attack the mineralized tooth cement. Strongly mineralized teeth, a result of inheritance and the mother's pregnancy diet, may provide resistance to these acids to some extent: but many children's teeth do nevertheless become decayed. For toddlers, the most cariogenic (caries-forming) foods are those that both contain sugar and get stuck between the teeth – some teething biscuits, sticky sweets, cakes, and cookies – and sweetened fruit drinks that bathe the teeth for long periods in a sugary solution.

The trouble is that sweet foods have become so loaded with symbolic meanings. Most parents and grandparents have at times used sugar to convey kindness, comfort, reassurance, and reward, and this symbolism can last a lifetime. In our household, which currently swarms with three-to-seven-year-olds, sugary foods make fairly frequent appearances. But they also disappear quickly, and we do not keep a store of them. In our view, total prohibition tends to create secret longings. While you still have control over what your toddler eats, we suggest you avoid giving him sugary foods. As he comes more and more in contact with the sugar-eating (and sugar-offering) world, try to find a happy balance. Introduce him to the toothbrush as soon as there are teeth to brush. And check that label! Don't be tempted to buy too many processed foods that contain sugar, sucrose, glucose, glucose syrup, dextrose or invert sugars: they all mean *sugar*.

When you do offer your child cake and cookies,

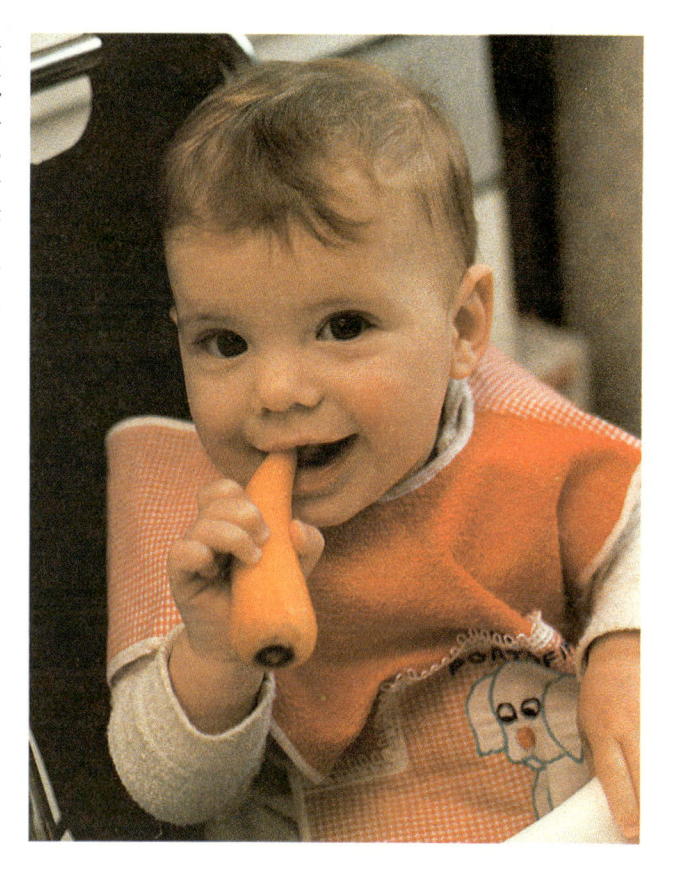

An early and delicious introduction to fresh produce.

because to deny them to him altogether may mean that he will come to seek them out all the more when outside the home, try to provide those that are not oversweet. Look out for recipes that do not feature sugar but are still delicious.

Sugarless muffins

2 cups flour, wholewheat
2 teaspoons baking powder
¼ cup sunflower oil
¼ cup honey
1¼ cups milk
1 egg

1. Combine the dry ingredients (flour and baking powder) in a small bowl.
2. Combine the wet ingredients (sunflower oil, honey, milk and egg) in a large bowl.
3. With a wooden spoon, fold the dry ingredients into the other bowl until the flour is just moistened.
4. Spoon the moist mixture into a well-greased muffin tin.
5. Bake for 20 minutes in an oven preheated to 400° F.
6. Serve with water, fruit juice or milk to drink.

Illness and diet

Young children are prone to mild illnesses that come quickly, and that wear off within a few days. An early sign is often loss of appetite. The child refuses to eat and, if you encourage him beyond what his little body wants, he vomits up his food. A fever often develops within hours, his body heating up as it tries to fight off whatever is afflicting him.

Among the many metabolic changes that occur with fever is a release of Vitamin C from its storage place in the liver into the bloodstream, which carries it through the body to strengthen cells at risk. Simultaneously, iron and other minerals are withdrawn from the blood into the liver, thus establishing – it is thought – an unfavorable environment for bacteria that have entered the bloodstream.[1,2] But a fever is a self-healing process, not an illness in itself. In our experience, a slight fever that lasts two or three days, with your toddler eating next-to-nothing but drinking plenty of water, does not need to be brought down with aspirin or other drugs. It will be particularly wise to avoid giving aspirin in instances of suspected viral illnesses, because it can cause very serious complications. Simply keep him warm and offer water and ice cubes, or chunks of cool fresh fruit. If you are still breastfeeding, continue to offer the breast. Anxiety on your part may delay the healing process, so try to stay positive. Your reassuring presence is probably his best medicine. But if the fever persists, or other symptoms such as spots or diarrhea appear, do consult your doctor. It may be the prelude to a bout of measles, chickenpox, or some other infectious and very commonplace childhood disease.

As the fever recedes, your child's appetite will gradually return. The best food to offer at this stage is something from the past; for illness is often accompanied by regression, a stepping back to a former stage of development, so that your toddler may become quite baby-like again. If you are still breastfeeding, your milk will be the best food for your baby.

If he still gets a bottle, this will probably be what he wants, filled with warm milk, at first diluted. For the completely weaned baby, a fairly liquid preparation of cream of rice, cooked with water at first, not milk, is likely to be accepted. His digestion may be delicate, so fatty foods, including whole milk and butter, should be avoided for the next day or two. A lukewarm vegetable or chicken broth may also be welcome.

As he recovers from the illness, you can gradually build up the range of solid foods he was eating before. This is the convalescence period, and it also offers you the chance to improve your child's diet and to make it more balanced, if that seems to be necessary.

Feasting and fasting

Let him feast if he has a mind to! A small child has a fine sense of balance in the long run, and his body will tell him when to stop. Occasional outbursts of joyful overeating now can be a good insurance against compulsive gorging later. Nor should you worry that feasting will unbalance his diet. As we have seen from Clara Davis's experiments, a healthy toddler offered a wide range of natural foods will eventually balance his own diet.

However, if you sense that feasting *has* become habitual gorging, you may have to take a closer look at his diet. Compulsive overeating usually indicates some anxiety that the child cannot resolve directly, perhaps a feeling he has picked up from you or from whoever spends most time with him.

If he wants to fast, refusing food for a day or so, the same applies. Do not worry that he will harm himself. On the contrary, young children stop eating at times when we adults might well do the same but do not: when they are becoming ill or are emotionally upset, or simply do not feel like eating, having more important things to do. Try to avoid hovering over your child to get him to eat more when he does not really want it. And try not to be resentful if you have spent a lot of time and energy preparing what he now rejects. If he learns to eat out of duty, he may lose the knack of eating out of hunger as he grows older. In this respect, a child who eats out of duty is like the bottle-fed baby who was fed by the clock. Mothers (and fathers) who have never voluntarily gone without a meal sometimes find it hard to believe that not eating for a while is an excellent way to rectify an unbalanced state of health in their children.

Constipation and diarrhea

Both these conditions can have physical or emotional causes. Constipation is normally transient, and it can usually be relieved by a diet containing plenty of fiber. Whole grains, vegetables, and fruit, both fresh and dried, promote regular bowel movements. Prunes are a time-tested laxative. The frequent use of laxatives, either natural or pharmaceutical, is not a good idea. If your toddler is regularly constipated, even on a high-fiber diet, he may be anxious or upset.

Transient diarrhea, lasting one or two days, may be due to a mild infection, an isolated meal of indigestible food, or to some passing emotional upset. If the cause passes, recovery is normally rapid. Suitable foods during this time are cream of wheat or rice, made with water instead of milk; rice and vegetable purée (carrots and onions are easily digested), and vegetable soup. Buttermilk, either alone or with mashed, very ripe banana, is excellent. Eggs are mildly constipating and may therefore help slow down the passage of food through the intestine.

Persistent diarrhea may be associated with chronic infection and is commonly treated with antibiotics. Make sure your doctor has identified the infection, as some antibiotics alter the bowel bacteria and can actually make diarrhea worse. Oral salts (see page 67) should always be given to prevent dehydration. Well-nourished children usually recover quickly when the diarrhea tapers off and soon begin to eat well again.

In the Third World, diarrhea is a killer. It comes from a combination of undernutrition, reduced resistance to disease, and infection, and it leads to dehydration, which can be fatal. With antibiotics, vitamin therapy and intensive feeding, young children with chronic severe diarrhea can recover, but these facilities are sometimes hundreds of miles away. In many of these countries, there are programs for the rehabilitation of starving babies, in small rural clinics staffed by 'barefoot doctors', local people instructed in the fundamentals of community medicine. But some forty thousand children still die *every day* in the Third World, over half of them as a result of infection and diarrhea.

Diarrhea also occurs under quite different circumstances, not as a result of infection or malnutrition but as an allergic reaction. Among babies, allergy to the proteins in cows' milk is relatively common; and in weaning, allergy to other foods, as they are introduced into the diet, may also present itself.

Food allergy

As your toddler comes into contact with new foods, new things and new places, he may turn out to be allergic to one or other of them. Allergy (from the Greek, meaning 'altered response') is the body's reaction to something it cannot tolerate (the *allergen*). It may be something in the air or in food, in drugs, or a substance that comes into contact with the skin. Some sufferers find that physical symptoms can even develop in the company of certain individuals, so that *people* can be allergenic too.

When symptoms occur, it is in at least one of four systems of the body: in the digestive tract, in the respiratory system, on the skin and in behavior. Food allergies may bring about symptoms in all of them.[3] However, when the symptoms first occur, it can be very hard to discover exactly what is causing them, because the reaction may come on many hours after exposure to the allergen. Thus it often requires very careful investigation before the problem substance is correctly identified.

There are many foods that can cause allergic reactions in susceptible toddlers. Wheat proteins (glutens), for example, cannot be tolerated by those with *celiac disease*, which obliges some children to go on a gluten-free diet for all their early years and sometimes for the rest of their lives. Milk proteins cannot be tolerated by some babies, and such an allergy may extend into childhood. Other common foods that can be allergenic include corn, pork, fish, onions, carrots, cabbage, cheese and other milk products, eggs, strawberries, raspberries, nuts, oranges, cocoa, chocolate, tea, and coffee.

Allergy to food additives has also been reported among young children. Dr. Ben Feingold has postulated a relationship between food additives, particularly artificial flavors and coloring, and hyperactivity in children, a condition that includes difficulties in perception, coordination, learning and social behavior.[4] Since 1973, he has conducted a dietary program in which affected children are given a diet free of artificial coloring and flavors, as well as all foods containing a natural salicylate compound related to aspirin. This last group include almonds, apples, apricots, cherries, cloves, currants, cucumbers, pickles, green peppers, mint, nectarines, oranges, peaches, plums, prunes, tomatoes, tangerines, tea, berries, grapes and raisins. Aspirin-related drugs are also excluded. Feingold claims a fifty percent response rate among hyperactive children. But as the treatment puts the child at the center of the family's attention, and hyperactive behavior is sometimes thought to be a direct response to inadequate attention, it is difficult to assess the importance of these findings. Controlled clinical trials of the effects of food additives on behavior are currently underway in Europe and the United States, though it is likely to be many years before we have a clear picture.

If your baby seems to be allergic to something, you will need to do a little detective work. A rash on his bottom could, for example, be due to the detergent in which you wash his diapers, to the diaper itself, to a cream, or to something in his urine or excrement, in turn derived from his diet. If you think you know the answer, test it by removing the suspected cause.

If the symptom disappears, you could be right. When allergy testing is properly done, the suspected allergen is replaced once the symptoms have cleared, to see if they return. If they do, the allergen is, if possible, removed from the baby's life. When the symptoms are causing the child distress – as they would be in persistent diarrhea, asthma, or eczema – you will need to see your doctor. These disorders can all have a wide range of nondietary causes.

Dietary deficiencies

Whenever children do not get a balanced diet, malnutrition may occur. At first, the effects are subtle. They may be nothing more than a loss of energy, a rash, a stiffness of the joints, a bout of coughing, or indigestion. Later, the signs may become more apparent, culminating in the full-blown clinical picture of deficiency disease. The signs of frank deficiency are easy to recognize, but those of milder deficiency are not.

Vitamin A deficiency is relatively common in very poor communities of the Third World, where it is the leading cause of blindness in preschool children. It frequently occurs as part of the under-nutrition syndrome called 'protein-energy malnutrition'. At first there is night blindness: difficulty in seeing in a dimly lit place where others can see reasonably well. Then the conjunctiva of the eyes become dry and dull, with foamy white spots forming towards the outer side of the iris. Finally the eyes ulcerate. The best protection is to eat plenty of Vitamin A-rich foods: carrots, sweet potatoes, egg yolk, and butter or fortified margarine, for example.

Vitamin D deficiency used to be common in the narrow sunless streets of industrial cities until cod-liver oil became a standard vitamin supplement earlier this century. Young children lacking both sunlight and a dietary source of the vitamin tend to develop rickets, with seizures, swollen wrists, fractures due to poor bone development, and a characteristic bowing of the legs. Manufactured in the skin on the action of sunlight, Vitamin D is also found in fish liver oils, fatty fish like tuna and mackerel, egg yolks, and lard.

Rickets is now relatively rare in the West, although it does still occur among the children of dark-skinned families who are genetically adapted to a lot of sunlight and who thus seem to need a lot of Vitamin D. A recent study of Indian children living in the British city of Bradford reported nearly half the toddlers with low Vitamin D levels in their blood and one in ten toddlers with overt rickets.[1] For children who see little of the sun, especially if they may be genetically adapted to a lot of sunlight, regular doses of cod-liver oil are recommended.

In the United States, most margarines and milk are enriched with synthetic Vitamin D, so that some children eat relatively large quantities of it. Experiments with animals have shown that high doses of Vitamin D can cause calcification of the blood vessels, for Vitamin D controls calcium metabolism; and it has been suggested that Vitamin D enrichment may be a cause of the relatively high incidence of atherosclerosis among young children.[2] A definite causal relationship between hardening of the arteries in childhood and eating too much enriched milk and margarine, whether eaten by the mother in pregnancy, or given to the young child, has yet to be proven. But one thing is certain: if your toddler does get these enriched foods, he will not need additional supplements of Vitamin D.

Vitamin C deficiency is probably more common than that of A or D, because this vitamin is stored only in relatively small amounts in the body and is rapidly used up in stress. Mild deficiency develops within three months if a baby is weaned to a diet very poor in fresh fruits and vegetables. The early symptoms are weakness, loss of appetite, and in some cases a run of illnesses as the child's resistance falls. In more extreme cases, the knees and ankles become swollen, and the skin rough and pale with bleeding spots. At this mature stage, the disease is known as *scurvy*. It is a most unpleasant looking and distressing condition when severe.

Including fresh fruits and vegetables in the diet will prevent scurvy, but in times of stress, whether physical (cold weather or mild illness, perhaps) or emotional (such as the birth of a sister or brother), additional Vitamin C is advisable to prevent mild deficiency. Hot lemon and honey (squeeze half a lemon into a cup, add a teaspoon of honey, and half fill the cup with hot water) is useful for colds and flu. At the first sign of a cold, you could also try giving your toddler 200 milligrams of Vitamin C powder. This may help to relieve the symptoms.

Iron deficiency, defined as a blood hemoglobin concentration below 11 grams per deciliter, is reported to be common among toddlers. Surveys of American preschool children show that ten percent of all one-to-six year olds, and twenty percent of those from poor families, are anemic by this standard. Measurement of the iron-binding capacity of the blood, another standard for assessing iron status, indicates that as many as forty-five percent may be at risk of iron deficiency.[3,4] The most commonly quoted cause of this phenomenon is weaning to a diet of foods containing inadequate iron. Whole grains, eggs, meat and fish, as well as dark leafy vegetables, remember, are good sources.

Iron deficiency can also be caused by drinking a lot of milk. Cows' milk contains very little iron; and the more of it a toddler drinks, the less he is likely to get of other iron-rich foods. A high milk intake – many toddlers are encouraged to drink as much as two pints a day – is also reported to damage the walls of the intestines in susceptible young children, causing blood loss, and therefore iron loss, in their stools. A pint of milk a day, whether taken straight from a cup or mixed into cooked dishes, is ample for a two-year-old, and half this amount is usually adequate.

Zinc deficiency – that is, abnormally low blood zinc levels – may also be widespread, though

Dietary deficiencies

without any apparent symptoms of illness or the poor growth that occurs in severe zinc deficiency.[5] White spots on the nails are said to be a good indicator and the cause is generally considered to be dietary. Eating a lot of sugar and white flour foods can lead to deficiency in a number of vitamins and minerals, including zinc, together with a relative excess of other minerals, such as copper and cadmium. A low ratio of zinc-to-copper and zinc-to-cadmium has been reported in the blood of adult cancer and heart disease patients,[6] and it has been suggested that a highly refined diet is a contributory cause.[7] There is no direct evidence, however, that this is the case.

According to Dr. Henry Schroeder of the Dartmouth Medical School in Vermont, the zinc to cadmium ratio is further unbalanced by a vast increase in environmental cadmium during the last thirty years, especially from the residues of cadmium fertilizers in the soil. This, according to Schroeder, is all the more reason for zinc intake to be maintained at a high level.[7]

There is evidence, too, that iron supplements may compete with zinc for absorption, and perhaps therefore contribute to zinc deficiency.[6] So convinced is the American Academy of Pediatrics that American children are not getting enough zinc that they have recommended that children's breakfast cereals (which are usually made from refined carbohydrates) should be enriched with zinc.[8] If you give your toddler a balanced wholefood diet, however, with whole grain breakfast cereals instead of the highly processed ones, he will not need zinc-enriched products. Zinc-rich foods include sunflower and pumpkin seeds, meat, cheese, herring, shellfish, and brewer's yeast.

Iodine is needed for the normal functioning of the thyroid gland and deficiency may lead to goitre, with its characteristic swelling of the throat, where the gland is located. Iodized salt has been widely available for many years and is commonly used, even where food comes from soil containing adequate iodine.

Fluoride is required for healthy bone and tooth formation, and fluoridation of tap water in low fluoride areas has been widely adopted to help combat rampant tooth decay among children. Several studies have shown that if one part fluoride is added to every million parts of drinking water, up to a fifty percent reduction in dental caries can occur. But recent research also now shows that this is too high a level of fluoridation for young babies.[9] Bottle-fed babies who receive formula made up with fluoridated water tend to develop *fluorosis*, a condition that stains the teeth and may adversely affect bone development. The American Academy of Pediatrics has now therefore reduced the recommended fluoridation level for infants to 0.25 parts per million.[9] This means that heavily fluoridated tap water can no longer be considered suitable for bottle-feeding; and in fluoridated areas, it is probably best for mothers to use bottled water. In contrast, fluoridation appears to have no effect on breastfeeding: breast milk fluoride levels remain constant, irrespective of the tap water content.

For toddlers aged from eighteen months to three years, the American Academy of Pediatrics recommends a fluoride intake of 0.5 mg. per day: and some authorities believe that this should be given in the form of a supplement. Tiny pills can be obtained on prescription. However, our children were not given such tablets, nor was their water fluoridated, yet their teeth are excellent. In our view, keeping sugar and other highly refined foods in the diet to an absolute minimum, and regular brushing with a fluoride toothpaste, are sound ways of ensuring that your child develops healthy teeth.

Teach your child good nutrition by letting him help you whenever possible in the kitchen.

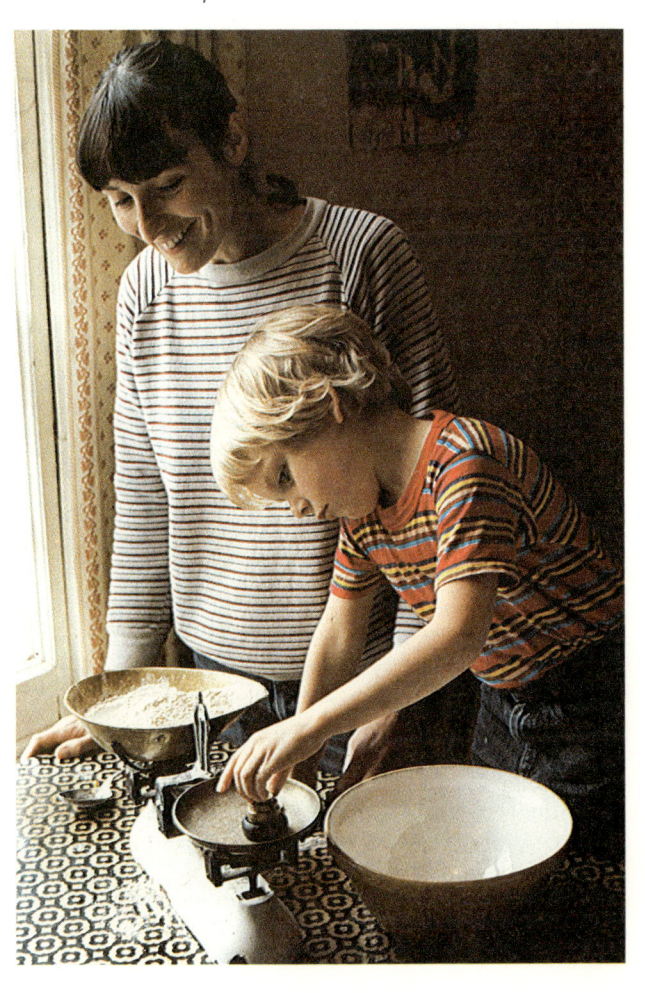

Supplements, rhythms and routines

Routine supplements for toddlers of vitamins (notably A, C, and D) and of minerals (particularly iron, zinc and fluoride) are recommended by some authorities. In general, the medical profession does not recommend them, while the market-place of popular nutrition has adopted them as essential. This has, of course, produced a boom for the vitamin manufacturers. Adelle Davis, a great advocate of routine supplements, convinced a whole generation of mothers, through her book *Let's Have Healthy Children*,[1] that routine supplementation is indispensible for good health. For several reasons, however, we find this view exaggerated.

Vitamin and mineral supplements are undoubtedly valuable in the treatment of certain well-defined nutritional disorders. Nor is there any doubt that a toddler raised on hot dogs, potato chips, and ice cream is likely to need regular vitamin and mineral supplements if he is to avoid deficiency.

But to say, as some authorities do, that all toddlers need daily supplements is to make a nonsense of their need to survive without pills in the long run. Anything taken habitually evokes some adaptation in our bodies so that, in time, we come to *need* it and cannot manage without it.

There are those who claim that the world has become so affected by technology that we can no longer expect to live well without taking supplements. The lead content of the atmosphere has, they say, increased five hundred times over the last thousand years;[2] and there is evidence from animal experiments that Vitamin C, as well as iron and zinc, provide some protection against lead poisoning by combining with it in the body and rendering it harmless. On these grounds, it has been argued that one should take routine, and sometimes massive supplements of Vitamin C, iron and zinc as insurance against environmental lead poisoning. But the evidence is very scanty, and the risks of routine supplementation are largely unknown. In our view, it is more sensible to eat plenty of *foods* containing those nutrients than to start a lifetime of pill-popping.

If, however, you do feel a need to give your toddler supplements, seek out those made from *natural* ingredients: for they tend to contain balances of nutrients similar to those that would be obtained from real food. Better still, use 'super-nutrient foods' like oranges and lemons which are loaded with Vitamin C; wheat germ, which is rich in Vitamin E, the B-Vitamins and iron; cod-liver oil which is very rich in Vitamins A, D, and E; and brewer's yeast with its high content of iron and zinc, as well as all the B-Vitamins. If your child eats meat, try liver from time to time; an animal's liver is its storehouse of many vitamins and minerals, but it is not essential to the diet.

It was commonly believed by our parents and grandparents that bottle-feeding was at least as good as breastfeeding: for a formula was said to contain everything a baby needed. But times have changed and now we know better. The breast milk of a well-nourished mother provides a far more appropriate food for her baby than any formula. Scientists, with all their technology, cannot make anything as good.

Perhaps the same is true of food in general. *Real, unrefined food*, as designed by the infinitely complex and wise processes of nature, can provide us with everything we need. Our survival as a species is the proof of it. Formulas are useful for babies who cannot get breast milk. Why not reserve supplements for children who cannot get a balanced diet of real food?

Getting into rhythm

Our lives and our bodies are permeated by invisible rhythms. Every twenty-four hours, for example, as the earth spins on its axis passing through a day and a night, our blood pressure rhythmically rises and falls. As the sun rises towards midday, the blood pressure rises; as the sun sets, the pressure falls. Our body temperature rises and falls in a similar twenty-four hour rhythm; and the same is true of the concentration in our blood of vitamins, amino acids, sugars, hormones and minerals, including zinc and iron. As every doctor knows, blood samples taken in the morning cannot be compared with samples taken in the afternoon, unless adjustments are made for these natural, rhythmical changes.

Natural rhythms also play an integral part in our growth, development and nutrition. In pregnancy, the fetus is nourished by his mother's rhythmically changing blood and – though such a thing has yet to be demonstrated – his growth probably responds in its own rhythmic way. The birth, too, is essentially a rhythmic affair, easily disrupted – as we have seen – by the routines of over-enthusiastic 'management'.[3]

The composition of breast milk also follows a twenty-four hour cycle. By the second week of life, once lactation has settled down, milk produced during the day is repeatedly lower in fat and greater in quantity than night milk, as though nature had especially prepared it for those hours when the baby has his greatest energy for sucking.[4] There is some evidence that the concentration of other nutrients in breast milk also follows a twenty-four hour rhythmic cycle. In contrast, the formula is utterly 'routine', retaining a constant composition, day and night.

The baby's hunger pattern is also rhythmic once feeding has settled down, provided that the mother responds to that hunger when it occurs, rather than feeding by the clock. In contrast, babies given bottles every four hours commonly fail to establish a hunger rhythm until after they are weaned: their own natural rhythms are overwhelmed by the routines imposed on them. The process is not, however, irreversible. Recent studies show that when a baby, once fed by the clock, is switched to demand-feeding, a natural rhythm rapidly emerges.[5]

As your baby grows, many of his biological rhythms change, so that, by about nine months, they are similar to those of his mother. This is the period during which the natural process of weaning develops, which emphasizes our view that weaning is properly speaking an integral part of the baby's physical and mental development. Not until between the sixth and ninth months, for example, does your baby develop a regular, twenty-four-hour rhythm for body temperature, blood sugar, urine composition, urine flow and heart rate:[6] which is to say that his body has taken six-to-nine months to adapt, at a very basic level, to life outside the womb. What is more, your baby's gradual adaptation to post-natal life is accompanied by changing nutritional requirements, and there is every reason to believe that weaning only becomes necessary when these requirements can no longer be met by the mother's milk. To disrupt the delicate timing of the physical, mental and nutritional process by introducing solids at four months, simply because this is the time recommended by many medical textbooks, is to ignore the true requirements of your baby.

In being sensitive to your baby's needs for food, comfort and affection, you are doing him a great service – enabling him to develop, both physically and emotionally, at his own pace and in his own way. A number of studies have shown that satisfactory weight gain by the end of the first year, and emotional stability (as measured by the ability of the baby to withstand short periods away from the mother) are strongly correlated to a mother's sensitivity to her baby's signals during feeding.[7,8] She loves him, attends to him, responds to him in the appropriate way: and he, in turn, responds to her sensitive attention by growing and developing in a healthy, happy way.

By his second year, your baby emerges from a world dominated by rhythms into one in which certain routines are now expected of him. If he and his rhythms have been respected up to now, the chances are that he will not find it hard to learn the art of respecting others. Mealtimes must gradually be fitted into family routines. He has to start learning how to use a potty. He is beginning to understand the word 'no'. The second year can be a terribly frustrating time if these developments are hurried along. Temper tantrums are not 'just one of those things that happen at this stage', but profound reactions to a clash between infantile rhythms and adult routines. The more you have respected his particular needs during the first year, the less trouble you will have now. As Dr. Donald Winnicott, the eminent British pediatrician, once wrote: "a mother's sensitive adaptation to her baby's needs starts off the idea (for the baby) of the world as a good place. The world goes to meet the infant and so the infant can go out to meet the world. The mother's cooperation with the baby at the beginning leads naturally on to the baby's cooperation with the mother".[9]

Sensitivity and the self-confidence to trust one's own intuitions are not, however, always easy qualities to nurture. Mothers sometimes ask: "How can I trust my own feelings about what to eat? How can I be sure that my milk will satisfy the baby? How will I ever know which foods to offer at weaning time? I need to be told these things". Health-care professionals all too often oblige by replying: "If you don't know what to eat in pregnancy, we will tell you. If you're afraid that you will not have sufficient milk for your baby, you can always use a formula. If you don't know when and how to wean, follow the routines in this brochure". Yet this kind of advice can draw a mother further and further away from following her baby's cues and her own intuition as to what is really needed. By all means, consult an 'expert' when something seems to be very wrong: but for day-to-day feeding, let your baby be your guide.

If you were fed by the clock as a baby or told to finish what was on your plate as a child, your attachment to these habits will be strong. As you feed your child, you will probably find yourself behaving just as your mother did, or your father or grandmother, re-enacting the same scenes you participated in so long ago. If it feels good and your baby is happy, fine. But if it feels wrong, and your baby seems not to be getting what he needs, experiment with something new. Let your child guide you through the possibilities. As you do so, a new way could emerge, not only about food and eating, but about life.

For the inventive, trusting, cheerful, spontaneous spirit of your child can open your eyes to a world you had forgotten: a world of great beauty and passion, pleasure and pain, a world of great intensity and infinite possibility. Nothing helps us more to reach into this place than shrinking to baby size, regressing for a while so as to see with a baby's eyes and take another look at life. Let your child fan the embers of your own inventive, trusting, cheerful, spontaneous spirit. Then you can grow together, your child for the first time and you for the second, or third . . .

Mother's nutrition notes

During child-bearing years, not only during pregnancy but also *prior* to conception and while breastfeeding, a balanced diet is all-important for both you and the baby. Use these two pages for your own nutrition notes, keeping a record of any supplements prescribed and their effects. For subsequent pregnancies, make copies of these pages and follow the same pattern.

Expected date of birth

Allergies
Suspected food	Date removed from diet	Effect

Supplements prescribed or recommended
Supplement (and brand)	Dose	Dates	Effects e.g. felt good, constipated, still tired etc.

Weight before and after birth

Start

1st month

2nd month

3rd month

4th month

5th month

6th month

7th month

8th month

term

immediately following the birth

six weeks after the birth

three months after the birth

six months after the birth

one year after the birth

Mother's nutrition notes

Pregnancy problems and pleasures
e.g. cravings, morning sickness, dreams, etc

Telephone numbers

Family doctor

Gynecologist/obstetrician

Pre-natal clinic

Pre-natal classes

Midwife (for home birth)

Hospital

Additional notes

Baby's nutrition notes

Whether you opt to breast or bottle-feed, your baby's nutrition is as important after the birth as it was before. Use these pages to record feeding progress, growth and weight gain, as well as a few details of the birth. Make copies of these pages to record details about other babies.

The birth

Date of birth (and time)

Place

Birth weight

The labor

When did it start?

How?

What did you do?

How was the birth?

Who was there?

Complications, if any

Feeding and sleeping patterns

Weaning

First new foods and dates

First meals and dates

Baby's nutrition notes

Weaning continued

Final breastfeeding (date)   Final bottle (if bottle-feeding)

Likes and dislikes

Food   Date   Comment

Allergies

Suspected food   Date removed from diet   Effect

Progress

Holds up head for a few seconds

Smiles

Laughs

Rolls over

Sits

Crawls

Stands up alone

First steps

First tooth

Out of diapers/day

Out of diapers/night

Sleeps through the night

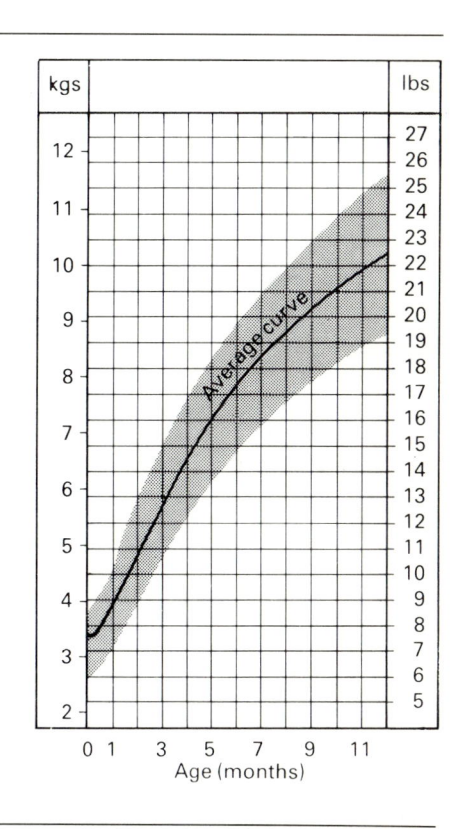

Average curve

kgs / lbs vs Age (months)

Telephone numbers

Breastfeeding counselor   Mother-and-baby groups

Baby clinic   Nutritionist

Baby sitter/helpful friends   Pediatrician

Glossary

Active birth a birth in which the mother is permitted and encouraged to deliver her infant in her own way, adopting the positions which are most comfortable to her during labor, perhaps standing or squatting for the birth itself.
Additives chemicals which are deliberately added to food in the manufacturing process, usually as preservatives or flavoring agents, or to modify texture.
Adrenal glands pea-sized *endocrine glands*, situated next to the kidneys, which have two distinct parts. The inner cortex produces *steroid hormones* which play many roles in metabolism: the outer medulla produces *adrenaline*, a hormone which prepares the body for extreme physical exertion.
Afterbirth see Placenta.
Allergen any substance capable of causing an *allergy*.
Allergy a sensitivity to substances such as pollen, plants, foods, dust or other normally harmless substances.
Alveoli the milk-secreting glands in the breasts.
Amino acids the building blocks of *proteins*. The 'essential' amino acids, of which there are ten, must be provided in the diet: the other 'non-essential' amino acids can be made by the body.
Amniotic fluid the fluid that surrounds the *fetus* in the *uterus*, also known as 'the waters'.
Amniotic sac the membrane containing the *amniotic fluid* that surrounds the fetus in the *uterus*: also known as the 'amnion' or 'bag of waters'.
Anemia insufficient *hemoglobin* in the blood, due either to a lack of the red blood cells which contain it, or to low levels of hemoglobin in these cells.
Anorexia loss of appetite.
Anorexic suffering from anorexia.
Antibodies proteins that the body produces in response to an *antigen* and which protect against infection.
Antigen anything that invades the body, often a micro-organism, and against which *antibodies* are formed.
Areola the pigmented area of skin that surrounds the nipple.
Ascorbic acid the chemical name for Vitamin C.
Atheroma the fatty degeneration of the inner layer of the arteries that is the beginning of *atherosclerosis*.
Atherosclerosis the progressive blocking up of the inside of the arteries, in regions where there is fatty degeneration. It is a cause of heart attacks and strokes.
Bile a thick yellow liquid secreted by the liver and stored in the gall-bladder. It has a function in digestion, particularly of fats, and contains waste materials thrown out by the liver.
Bilirubin a bile pigment, derived from red blood cells. *See also Bile, Jaundice.*
Blastocyst the early stage of the developing, newly fertilized *ovum*.
Bowel that part of the digestive system below the stomach, also known as the intestine.
Bran the broken outer covering of milled grains: a good source of *roughage* or dietary *fiber*.
Caesarian section delivery of a baby by surgical means, via the mother's abdomen.
Caffeine a stimulant which also has diuretic properties. It is found in coffee and tea, and in certain carbonated drinks, as well as being a constituent of some headache tablets.
Calcium an essential mineral and a constituent of bones and teeth. The chief dietary sources are milk, cheese, fish, and green vegetables.
Calorie a unit of energy: the amount of heat needed to raise the temperature of 1 kg of water by 1°C.
Carbohydrates energy-producing organic compounds, including the sugars and starches.
Caries tooth decay.
Catalyst a substance that speeds up a chemical reaction or makes possible one which would not otherwise occur. *See also Enzymes.*
Celiac disease a sensitivity to wheat or rye products, thought to be an allergy to the protein *gluten* found in them. It most often develops in the two years after weaning but may also suddenly appear for the first time in adult life.
Cervix the neck or lower part of the *uterus*, leading to the *vagina*.
Cholesterol a substance necessary for the formation of bile salts and certain hormones. The body can make its own cholesterol: but excess taken in with animal products is believed to promote *atherosclerosis*.
Chromosomes the nucleus of every human cell contains twenty-three pairs of these rod-like structures, which contain the *genes*.
Colic in infants, an attack of incessant convulsive screaming, probably due to abdominal pain but now also widely believed to be due to emotional causes.
Colostrum the first milk produced in the few days after birth. Rich in *antibodies*, it provides a certain degree of immunity to the baby.
Conception fertilization of the *ovum* by the *sperm* to form a *blastocyst* or fertilized *ovum*.
Congenital abnormality a deformity existing at birth, not necessarily hereditary.
Constipation irregular and difficult moving of the bowels.
Copper a mineral essential to a healthy diet in trace amounts. It is needed mainly for the formation of red corpuscles. Symptoms of deficiency include *anemia*.
Curds coagulated milk solids, mostly protein, and formed by the action of the gastric juices on milk.
Dehydration a fall in the amount of water in the body due to inadequate intake or excessive loss. Only a small degree of dehydration can be tolerated, particularly by small babies.
Diabetes (mellitus) a disease in which the body fails to metabolize glucose as it should, as a result of lack of insulin, causing excessively high levels of sugar in the blood and urine.
Diarrhea frequent watery bowel movements, which can be a serious condition in infants, because of loss of minerals and risk of dehydration.
Diuretic a drug that increases the amount of urine produced.
Down's syndrome a form of congenital abnormality involving mental deficiency, formerly known as *Mongolism*.
Eclampsia a severe form of *pre-eclampsia* with symptoms of high blood pressure, seizures and visual disturbances.
Eczema a non-infective inflammatory condition of the skin.
Edema a swelling of various parts of the body, particularly the hands or feet, due to fluid retention.
Embryo a term for the developing baby up to the seventh week of pregnancy. Thereafter, until birth, the baby is known as the *fetus*.
Endocrine glands glands in the body which produce *hormones*. Examples are the *pituitary*, *adrenal* and *thyroid* glands, as well as the *pancreas*.
Endosperm the inner part of the cereal grain, enclosed inside it with the *germ*.
Enzymes proteins which act as highly specific *catalysts* for all the chemical reactions in the body.
Enteric of the intestines.
Epidural a form of local *anesthesia* involving injection of an anesthetic into the epidural space which surrounds the spinal cord.
Episiotomy a surgical incision into the *perineum*, to enlarge the birth outlet, theoretically in order to facilitate delivery of the baby's head.
Fallopian tubes two tubes that run from the *ovaries* to the *uterus*, and down which the *ovum* passes. Conception occurs in the Fallopian tubes.
Fatty acids the building blocks of fats.
Fertilizers substances used to improve the ability of the soil to nourish plants.
Fetus the developing baby from the seventh week after conception until birth.
Fiber a component in the diet which is not digested to any great extent but is necessary to prevent constipation as well as being beneficial to general health.
Fluoride a form of the element fluorine which protects against tooth decay. It is often added to toothpaste and, in some areas, to tap water in the attempt to promote healthy teeth.
Fluorosis a condition affecting the teeth, with mottling of the enamel brought on by excessive fluoride intake.
Folic acid a vitamin of the B group, found in green vegetables, kidney, liver and yeast. Symptoms of folic acid deficiency can occur in pregnancy unless care is taken with the diet.
Formula an infant food intended as a substitute for breast milk, usually fortified with essential vitamins and minerals.
Galactosemia a rare disease in which an infant cannot convert *galactose*, the sugar derived from *lactose*, into *glucose*.
Gastroenteritis usually the result of an infection, an inflammation of the stomach and intestine with severe symptoms of *diarrhea* and vomiting.
Genes component parts of the chromosomes, and the means by which hereditary characteristics are passed on.
Germ in nutrition, that part of the cereal grain which contains the developing plant and which is a rich source of nutrients.
Glucose a simple sugar used as a fuel by the body. All other sugars can be converted into glucose in the body.
Gluten a protein found in various cereals, including wheat. *See Celiac disease.*

Glossary

Goitre an enlargement of the *thyroid gland*, in extreme cases visible as a large swelling in the neck, usually due to a diet lacking in *iodine*.
Gynecologist a doctor specializing in the female reproductive system. *See also Obstetrician.*
Hatha yoga an Indian system of meditative exercise and breathing; one of many forms of *yoga*.
Hemoglobin part of the red blood cells that contains iron. Its red color accounts for the color of the cells, and its function is to transport oxygen around the body.
Hemorrhage bleeding.
Hormones the chemical messengers of the body, produced by the *endocrine glands* and carried in the blood.
Hyperactivity activity exceeding the normal.
Hypertension high blood pressure.
Hypotension low blood pressure.
Immunity a resistance to infection.
Insulin a hormone secreted by the *pancreas*, and which controls the ability of cells to take up glucose from the blood.
Iodine an essential mineral found in many foods, especially seafood. An inadequate intake of iodine will cause goitre.
Iron an essential mineral and an important constituent of *hemoglobin*. Particularly good sources are nuts, meat, eggs, and liver.
Jaundice a condition in which the liver is immature or fails to work efficiently so that a substance known as *bilirubin* accumulates in the bloodstream, causing a yellow tinge to the skin.
Kidneys a pair of glands, situated at the back of the abdomen, the function of which is to produce urine.
Lactation the production of breast milk.
Lactose the sugar of milk, made from *glucose* and *galactose*.
Legume the pod or seed of a leguminous plant; peas and beans are examples. They are good sources of protein.
Liver a large organ in the abdomen involved in many activities including secreting *bile*, making *proteins*, breaking down poisons in the blood and making *glucose*.
Low-birth-weight baby a baby born weighing under five-and-a-half pounds at birth.
Macrobiotic diet a diet balanced according to the Chinese principles of *yin* and *yang*. Based on wholegrain cereals, it includes most vegetables, and fish, but very little meat, dairy produce and fruit; sugar is *taboo*.
Meconium the contents of the bowel of the fetus, excreted during the first days after the birth. Blackish-green and very sticky, it is mostly *bile* and mucus.
Metabolism the highly complex system of chemical reactions which supports life, and involves the body's use of nutrients.
Midwife a specially trained nurse responsible for care during labor and delivery.
Minerals the metal part of salts found in foods, many of which are needed in small amounts for good health.
Mongolism see *Down's syndrome*.
Naso-gastric tube a flexible tube passed into the stomach via the nose, which may be used for feeding or introducing medicines into the stomach, or to empty the stomach. Premature babies are sometimes fed in this way.
Natural childbirth childbirth in which there is minimal medical intervention.
Nutrients components of food necessary for growth and the maintenance of good health.
Obstetrician a doctor specializing in the care of women during pregnancy and birth.
Ovaries the two female glands from which one egg or *ovum* is usually released each month.
Ovum the female egg cell.
Oxytocin a hormone produced by the *pituitary gland* which controls uterine contractions and milk production. An artificial form is used to stimulate contractions of the *uterus* when delivery is induced.
Pancreas the gland situated below and behind the stomach and liver, secreting the hormone *insulin* into the blood and the intestines, where it helps digestion.
Pediatrician a doctor specializing in the care of babies and small children.
Pica cravings for substances that are not actually food, like coal or dirt. They sometimes occur in pregnancy and in young children.
Pituitary gland a small endocrine gland at the base of the brain that influences growth and various bodily functions by producing *oxytocin* and *prolactin*, among other hormones.
Placenta an organ in the womb which unites mother to fetus. It is delivered after the baby is born and then is known as the *afterbirth*.
Pre-eclampsia a pregnancy condition, also known as *toxemia of pregnancy*, involving nausea, high blood pressure, water retention and loss of protein in the urine.
Premature birth after a short gestation period (usually before thirty-seven weeks). Premature or pre-term babies are normally of low birth weight (under five-and-a-half pounds). They are usually distinguished from low birth weight babies who are born full-term.
Prolactin the *hormone* which initiates *lactation*.
Proteins the major building blocks of the cells of the body and thus an essential part of the diet. Made from *amino acids*, proteins are found in both plant and animal foods.
Rickets a childhood disease due to Vitamin D deficiency, with a characteristic softening of the bones, visible as bowing of the legs and enlarged joints.
Roughage food, such as wheat bran, fruit or fibrous meat, which is said to prevent constipation and may also confer other health benefits.
Scurvy a deficiency disease due to lack of Vitamin C, in which connective tissue of the gums and skin breaks down.
Sodium an essential mineral provided by many foods and the salt we add to them.
Sperm the male reproductive cells, one of which must fertilize the female egg for conception to occur.
Thyroid the endocrine gland in the neck that regulates the rate at which the body burns food and which is also part of the mechanism controlling the rate of growth.
Umbilical cord the threefold cord which connects the developing baby to the *placenta*. It comprises a vein and two arteries.
Uterus a woman's womb, the normally pear-shaped hollow muscle in which the fetus develops. It is connected by the *Fallopian tubes* to the *ovaries*, and via the *cervix* to the *vagina*.
Vagina the passage leading, in a woman, from the *vulva* to *cervix*. It is also called the birth canal.
Villi short hair-like protrusions on the walls of the intestines, giving it a velvety texture. Digested food is absorbed by the villi into the blood.
Vitamins a group of chemical substances found in food, essential in tiny quantities for healthy growth and development. They are commonly identified by letters and sometimes numbers, too.
Weaning the process in which milk is gradually replaced in the baby's diet by non-milk foods, as part of the baby's developing independence from the mother.
Whey the watery part of the milk left after curds are formed. *See also Curds.*
Yang according to Eastern medicine and philosophy, the active or male principle or force in nature, characterized by heating, drying and contracting. *See also Yin.*
Yeast a micro-organism used in the making of bread and in the brewing of beer. It contains high concentrations of the B Vitamins and is sometimes used as a dietary supplement.
Yin the passive or female principle or force in nature, according to Oriental tradition, characterized by cooling, moistening and expanding. *See also Yang.*
Yoga literally meaning 'union', a system of meditations and exercises, practiced daily to promote well-being. *See also Hatha Yoga.*
Zen macrobiotics See *Macrobiotic diet.*
Zinc a mineral which, although needed only in trace amounts, is essential to good health.

Cookbooks

Creative, attractive wholefood cookbooks can be found by the dozens in most large bookstores. Look for those that suit your lifestyle. To get you started, watch for the following, recommended by the publisher:

As You Eat, So Your Baby Grows by Nikki and David Goldbeck (New American Library, 1977)
The Book of Whole Meals by Annemarie Colbin (Ballantine, 1983)
Eating Naturally by Maggie Black and Pat Howard (Faber and Faber, 1980)
Eating Right for Two: The Complete Nutrition Guide and Cookbook for a Healthy Pregnancy by Diane Klein and Rosalyn Badalamenti (Ballantine, 1983)
Feed Me, I'm Yours by Vicki Lansky (Meadowbrook, 1980)
Making Your Own Babyfood by James Turner (Bantam, 1978)
Mother Earth's Vegetarian Feasts by Joel Rapp (William Morrow & Co., 1984)
Natural Babyfood by Brenda O'Casey (Duckworth, 1977)
The Natural Foods Primer by Beatrice Trum Hunter (Simon & Schuster, 1972)
The New York Times New Natural Foods Cookbook by Jean Hewitt (Times Books, 1982)
Rodale's Basic Natural Foods Cookbook edited by Charles Gerras (Rodale, 1984)
The Rodale Cookbook by Nancy Albright (Ballantine, 1982)

References

Abbreviations
ADC Archives of Diseases in Childhood: AJCN American Journal of Clinical Nutrition: AJDC American Journal of Diseases in Childhood: AJE American Journal of Epidemiology: AJN American Journal of Nursing: AJOG American Journal of Obstetrics and Gynecology: APS Acta Paediatrica Scandinavica: BJ Biochemical Journal, London: BJH British Journal of Haemotology: BJOG British Journal of Obstetrics and Gynaecology: BMJ British Medical Journal: BP Behavioural Processes: BR Bacteriological Review: CMAJ Canadian Medical Association Journal: CMJ Chinese Medical Journal: CMRO Current Medical Research Opinion: CS Clinical Obstetrics and Gynaecology: CS Clinical Science: DMCN Developmental Medicine and Child Neurology: DP Developmental Psychobiology: FP Federation Proceedings: IDJ International Dental Journal: IJMS Israeli Journal of Medical Science: IJVNR International Journal for Vitamin and Nutrition Research: JACS Journal of The American Cancer Society: JAMA Journal of the American Medical Association: JEM Journal of Experimental Medicine: JHN Journal of Human Nutrition: JID Journal of Infectious Diseases: JMG Journal of Medical Genetics: JN Journal of Nutrition: JOG Journal of Obstetrics and Gynaecology: JTP Journal of Tropical Pediatrics: L Lancet: LLI La Leche League International: MH Medical Hypotheses: MJA Medical Journal of Australia: MO Medical Officer: NEJM New England Journal of Medicine: NRI Nutrition Reports International: NS New Scientist: NT Nutrition Today: NZJS New Zealand Journal of Science: OG Obstetrics and Gynecology: P Pediatrics: PCNA Pediatric Clinics of North America: PMJ Postgraduate Medical Journal, Oxford: PNS Proceedings of the Nutrition Society: PR Physiological Reviews: PS Population Studies: PSEBM Proceedings of the Society for Experimental Biology and Medicine: RSHJ Royal Society of Health Journal: S Science: SAMJ South African Medical Journal: SMJ Southern Medical Journal, Birmingham.

Conception
(pages 8–9)
1. Newton N (1977) The role of oxytocin reflexes in the three interpersonal reproductive acts. *In* Proceedings of the 1976 Serono Symposium on Clinical Psycho-Neuroendocrinology etc. Ed: Zichella L, Academic Press, UK. **2.** Smith CA (1947) The effect of wartime starvation in Holland upon pregnancy. AJOG, 53:599. **3.** Stein Z, Susser M, Saenger G, Marola F (1975) Famine and Human Development: the Dutch Hunger Winter 1944-5. Oxford University Press, New York. **4.** Drillen CM (1957) Social and economic factors affecting the incidence of premature birth. JOG, 64:161. **5.** Cravioto J, et al (1966) Nutrition, growth and neuro-intergrative development. P, 38:319. **6.** Gruenwald P (1975) The placenta and its maternal supply line. MTP Press, Aylesbury, UK. **7.** Wynn M, Wynn A (1977) Prevention of preterm birth. Foundation for Education and Research in Childbearing, UK. **8.** Bresler DE, et al (1975) Learning deficits in rats with malnourished grandmothers. DP, 8 (4):315. **9.** Zamenhof S (1971) S, 72:850. **10.** Hurley LS (1980) Development Nutrition. Prentice-Hall Inc, New Jersey. **11.** Lindner E (1958) Therapeutische Bedeutung des Vitamin E. Internationale Zeitschrift fur Vitaminforsch, 29:33. **12.** Hartoma T, et al (1977) Zinc plasma, androgens and male sterility, 2:1125. **13.** Suzuki T, Yoshida A (1979) JN, 109:1974. **14.** Johnson NE, Tenuta K (1979) Diets and blood levels of children who practice pica. Environmental Research, New York, 18:369. **15.** Cerklewski FL (1979) Influence of dietary zinc on lead toxicity during gestation and lactation in the female rat. JN, 109:1703. **16.** Suzuki T, Yoshida A (1979) Effect of dietary supplementation of iron and ascorbic acid in the prevention and cure of moderately long-term lead toxicity in rats. JN, 109:1974. **17.** Stolkowski J, Choukroun J (1981) IJMS, 17:1061. **18.** Dhanaraj VH (1974) The effects of yoga and the 5BX Fitness Plan on selected physiological parameters. University of Alabama. **19.** Kishi H (1977) Deficiency of Vitamin B_6 in women taking oral contraceptives. Research Communications in Chemical Pathology and Pharmacology, Westbury, New York, 17:283. **20.** Roepke, JLB, Kirsey A (1974) Vitamin B_6 nutriture during pregnancy and lactation. AJCN, 32:2249. **21.** Applegate WW, et al (1979) Physiological and psychological effect of Vitamins E and B_6 on women taking oral contraceptives. IJVNR, 49:43. **22.** Roe DA (1976) Nutritional effects of oral contraceptives *in* Drug-induced nutritional deficiencies. Ed: Roe DA, AVI Publishing, Westport, 247–252.

From embryo to fetus
(pages 10–11)
1. Longo LD (1972) Placental transfer mechanisms – an overview. Obstetrics and Gynecology Annual, New York, 1:103. **2.** Mott FJ (1959) The nature of the self: the human mind rediscovered in a specific instance of universal configuration governing all integration. Allan Wingate, UK. **3.** Levi-Strauss C (1966) The Savage Mind. Weidenfeld and Nicholson, UK. **4.** Mistretta CM, Bradley RM (1975) Taste and swallowing in utero. British Medical Bulletin, 31(1):8. **5.** de Snoo K (1937) Das trinkende Kind im Uterus. Monatsschrift fur Geburtshilfe und Gynakologie, Berlin, 105:88. **6.** Verny T, Kelly J (1982) The secret life of the unborn child. Sphere Books, UK.

Diet in pregnancy
(pages 12–13)
1. Mellanby E (1933) Nutrition and Childbearing. L, 1131. **2.** Ebbs JH, Tisdall FF, Scott WA (1941) Influence of pre-natal diet on mother and child. JN, 22:515. **3.** Burke BS, et al (1943) Nutrition studies during pregnancy. JOG, 46:38. **4.** Balfour MI (1944) PNS, 2:27. **5.** Higgins AC (1973) Montreal Diet Dispensary Study. *In* Nutritional supplementation and the outcome of pregnancy. US National Academy of Science. **6.** Rush D (1981) Nutrition services during pregnancy and birth weight: a retrospective matched pair analysis. CMAJ, 125:567. **7.** Davidson S, et al (1979) Human nutrition and dietetics. Churchill Livingstone, UK. **8.** UK Department of Health (1976) Research on Obesity: a report of the DHSS/MRC Group. HMSO, London. **9.** Ounsted MK, Simons CD (1976) Infant feeding, growth and development. CMRO, 4 (Suppl. 1):60. **10.** Wright P, et al (1980) The development of the difference in the feeding behaviour of bottle and breastfed infants. BP, 5:1. **11.** Gunther M, Stanier JE (1949) Diurnal variation in the fat content of breast milk. L, 2:235. **12.** Ashworth A (1974) Ad Lib feeding during recovery from malnutrition. BJN, 31:109. **13.** Davis C (1939) Results of the self-selection of diets by young children. CMAJ, 4:257. **14.** Schachter S (1973) Obesity and eating: internal-external cues differentially affect the early eating behaviour of obese and normal subjects. S, 161:751. **15.** Hamburger WW (1960) Appetite in Man. AJCN, 8:596.

Guidelines for a balanced diet
(pages 14–23)
1. FAO (1977). World Food Survey. Food and Nutrition Series No. 10. **2.** Schwab MG (1973) Bread in Man's Diet, MSc (Nutrition) thesis, London University. **3.** McCarrison R (1945) Studies in deficiency disease. Oxford Medical Publications, Frowde and Hodder & Stoughton, London. Reproduced by The Lee Foundation, Milwaukee. **4.** Price WA (1939) Nutrition and physical degeneration: a comparison of primitive and modern diets and their effects. Paul Hoeber, New York. **5.** Brusis OA, McGandy RB (1971) Risk factors in coronary heart disease. FP, 30:1417. **6.** Walker ARP (1948) Studies in human mineral metabolism. BJ, 42:452. **7.** Turner RWD (1980) Coronary heart disease: the size and nature of the problem. *In* Dietary prevention of coronary heart disease. Eds: Ball, KP, Turner RWD. PMJ, 56:658. **8.** Crawford M, Crawford S (1972). What we eat today. Neville Spearman, UK. **9.** Swann MM (1969) Chairman Joint Committee on the Use of Antibiotics in Animal Husbandry. HMSO, London. **10.** FAO/WHO (1977) Dietary fats and oils in human nutrition. **11.** FAO (1977) World Food Survey. Food and Nutrition Series No 10. **12.** Ohsawa G (1965) Zen Macrobiotics. Ohsawa Foundation, San Francisco. **13.** Yudkin J (1972) Pure White and Deadly. Davis-Poynter, UK. **14.** Cleave TL, et al (1969) Diabetes, coronary thrombosis and the saccharine disease. John Wright, UK. **15.** United Kingdom (1955) Food and Drugs Act. HMSO, London. **16.** TACC, Technology Assessment Consumerism Centre (1975) Bread. Intermediate Publishing, UK. **17.** Gross D (1977) Our polluted food – fact or fancy? RSHJ, 5:193. **18.** Mohr U, et al (1966) Cancer Research 26:2349. **19.** Yudkin J (1976) This Nutrition Business. Davis-Poynter, UK. **20.** Cahill MA (1982) Environmental contaminants in breast milk. LLI Information Sheet No. 82. **21.** Lesser M (1980) Nutrition and Vitamin therapy. Grove Press. **22.** Cohen AM, et al (1961)L, 2:1939.

Dietary taboos and dangers
(pages 24–25)
1. Wilson CS (1980) Food taboos of childbirth. *In* Food, Ecology and Culture. Ed: Robson JRK. Gordon & Breach. **2.** Storer J (1977) Hot and cold beliefs in an Indian community and their significance. JHN, 31:33. **3.** Das R (1972) India's food and nutrition problems. *In* Perspectives in Nutrition, University of Baroda. Cited in Storer J (1977) *above*. **4.** Rhead WJ, Schrauzer GN (1971) Risks of long-term ascorbic acid overdosage. Nutrition Reviews, New York, 11:262. **5.** Levi-Stauss C (1966) The Savage Mind. Weidenfeld and Nicholson, London. **6.** Ouelette EM, et al (1977) Adverse effects on offspring of maternal alcohol abuse. NEJM, 297:528. **7.** Turner G (1978) Ed: The fetal alcohol syndrome. MJA, 1:18. **8.** Fox HE, et al (1978) Maternal ethanol ingestion and the occurrence of human fetal breathing movements. AJOG, 132:354. **9.** Blake DA (1982) Risks of alcohol in pregnancy. *In* Drug use in pregnancy. Ed: Niebyl JR. Lea and Febiger, Philadelphia. **10.** Kline JL et al (1980) Drinking during pregnancy and spontaneous abortion L, 2:176. **11.** Streissguth AP (1978) Fetal alcohol syndrome: an epidemiologic perspective. AJE, 107:467. **12.** Heinonen OP, et al (1977) Caffeine and other xanthine derivatives. *In* Birth defects and drugs in pregnancy. Publishing Services Group Inc. Littleton, Mass. **13.** Nelson MM, Forfar JO (1971) Associations between drugs administered during pregnancy and congenital abnormalities of the fetus. BMJ, 1:523. **14.** Lechtat MF, et al (1980) Caffeine Study (letter) S, 207:1296. **15.** Lust JB (1978) The Herb Book. Bantam Books. **16.** Meyer MB (1982) Smoking and pregnancy. *In* Drug use in pregnancy Ed: Nebyl JR. Lea and Febiger, Philadelphia. **17.** Crosby WM, et al (1977) Fetal malnutrition: an appraisal of correlated factors. AJOG, 128:22. **18.** Lehtovirta P, Forss M (1978) The acute affect of smoking on intervillous blood flow of the placenta. BJOG, 85:729. **19.** Hasselmeyer EG, et al (1980) Pregnancy and infant health. *In* The health consequences of smoking women: a report of the Surgeon General. Health, Education and Welfare publication no. 637950069. **20.** Hickey RJ, et al (1978) Maternal smoking, birth weight, infant death and the self-selection problem. AJOG, 131:805. **21.** Rantakillio P (1978) The effect of maternal smoking on birth weight and subsequent health of the child. Early Human Development, Amsterdam,

References

4:371. **22.** Yerushalmy J (1972) Infants of low birth weight born before their mothers started to smoke cigarettes. AJOG, 112:277. **23.** Andrews J, McGarry JM (1972) A community study of smoking in pregnancy. JOG, 79:1057. **24.** Low CR (1959) Effect of mothers' smoking habits on birth weight of their children. BMJ, 2:673. **25.** Underwood P, et al (1965) The relationship of smoking to the outcome of pregnancy. AJOG, 91:270. **26.** Gritz ER (1978) Women and smoking: a realistic approach. *In* Progress in smoking cessation. JACS. **27.** Jacobson B (1981) Women: smoking's new victims. NS, 90:506. **28.** Ryan P, et al (1980) Experiences of pregnancy. Pregnant Pause Campaign. Div. Drugs & Alcohol Services, Health Commission of New South Wales.

The nutrients in pregnancy
(pages 26–27)

1. Hurley LS (1980) Developmental nutrition. Prentice-Hall, New Jersey. **2.** Osofsky HJ (1975) Relationships between perinatal medical and nutritional measures, pregnancy outcome and early infant development in an urban poverty setting. AJOG, 23:682. **3.** Rush D (1981) Nutrition services during pregnancy and birthweight: a retrospective matched pair analysis. CMAJ, 125:567. **4.** Higgins A (1974) A preliminary report of a nutrition study on public maternity patients. Report of a workshop on nutritional supplementation. National Research Council of 1972. **5.** Hornston G (1980) Effect of dietary fat on arterial thrombosis. *In* Ball KP, Turner WD (1980) Dietary prevention of coronary heart disease. PMJ, 56:563. **6.** DHSS (1974) Diet and coronary heart disease. Report on Health and Social Subjects No. 7. Department of Health and Social Security, UK. **7.** Hytten FE, Leitch I (1971) The physiology of human pregnancy. Blackwell Scientific Publications.

The micro-nutrients in pregnancy
(pages 28–31)

1. Smithells RW, Sheppard S (1980) Possible prevention of neural tube defects by peri-conceptual vitamin supplementation. 1:647. **2.** James WH (1981) Recurrence rates for neural tube defects and vitamin supplementation. JMG, 18(4):249. **3.** Medical Research Council (1982). Randomised clinical trial of folic acid and other vitamin supplementation in the prevention of neural tube defects. MRC Press Release, UK. **4.** Hurley LS (1980) Developmental Nutrition. Prentice-Hall, New Jersey. **5.** Roepke JLB, Kirsey A (1974) Vitamin B_6 nutriture during pregnancy and lactation. AJCN, 32:2249. **6.** Brook OG et al (1980) Vitamin D supplementation of pregnant Asian women: effects of calcium status and fetal growth. BMJ, 1:751. **7.** Kutsky RJ (1981) Handbook of vitamins, minerals and hormones. Van Nostrand Rheinhold, Cincinnati. **8.** Hemminki E, Starfield B (1978) Routine administration of iron and vitamins during pregnancy: review of controlled clinical trials. BJOG, 85:404. **9.** Averback P (1976) Anencephaly associated with megavitamin therapy. CMAJ, 14:95. **10.** Seller M et al (1974) Neural tube defects in curly tailed mice II: effects of maternal administration of Vitamin A. Proceedings of the Royal Society of London. Series B, 54:101. **11.** Neuweiler W (1951) Hypervitaminosis and its relation to pregnancy. Internationale Zeitschrift fur Vitaminforschung 22:392. **12.** Samborskaya EP (1966) Effect of large doses of ascorbic acid on pregnant guinea pigs. Bulletin of Experimental Biology and Medicine, Moscow, 57:105. **13.** Jakovlieu N (1958) Scurvy following nutritional stress. Ernaehrungsforschung 3:446. **14.** Rhead WJ, Schrauzer GN (1971) Risks of long-term ascorbic acid overdosage. Nutrition Reviews, New York, 11:262. **15.** Cochrane WA (1965) Overnutrition in prenatal and neonatal life: a problem? CMAJ, 93:893. **16.** Kutsky (1981) Handbook of vitamins, minerals and hormones. Van Nostran Rheinhold, Cincinnati. **17.** Widdowson EM (1977) Nutrition and lactation. Current Concepts in Nutrition, 5:67. **18.** Sheolikar IS (1970) Absorption of dietary calcium in pregnancy. AJCN, 23(1):63. **19.** Walker ARP, et al (1972) The influence of numerous pregnancies and lactations on bone dimensions in South African Bantu and Causasian mothers. CS, 42:189. **20.** Hammar M, et al (1981) Calcium treatment of leg cramps in pregnancy. Acta Obstetricia et Gynecologica Scandinavica, Stockholm, 60:345. **21.** Balfour WM, et al (1942) Radioactive iron absorption in clinical conditions etc. JEM, 76:15. **22.** Hahn PF, et al (1951) Iron metabolism in human pregnancy as studied with a radioactive isotope Fe59. AJOG, 61:477. **23.** Fenton V (1977) Iron stores in pregnancy. BJH, 37:145. **24.** Elsborg L, et al (1979) Iron intake by teenage girls and by pregnant women. IJVNR, 49:210. **25.** Hytten FE, Leitch I (1971) The physiology of human pregnancy, Blackwell. **26.** Money DLF (1978) Vitamin E, selenium, iron and Vitamin A content of livers from SIDS cases and control children. NZJS, 21:41. **27.** Forth W, Rummel W (1973) Iron absorption. Physiological Reviews 53:724. **28.** Momcilovic M, Kello D (1979) Fortification of milk with zinc and iron. NRI, 20:429. **29.** Taylor, DJ, Lind T (1976) Haematological changes during normal pregnancy: iron induced macrocytosis. BJOG, 83:760. **30.** WHO (1965) Report of the Expert Committee on Nutrition in Pregnancy and Lactation. **31.** Thomson AM (1976) Fetal Growth. *In* Early Nutrition and Later Development. Ed: Wilkinson AW. Pitman Medical, UK.

Energy, calories and weight gain
(pages 32–35)

1. Brewer G, Brewer T (1982) What every pregnant woman should know. AIMS Books, UK. **2.** Singer et al (1968) AJOG, 31:417. **3.** Shank RE (1970) A chink in our armour. NT, 5:2. **4.** Campbell DM, MacGillivray I (1976) The effect of a low-calorie or a thiazide diuretic on the incidence of pre-eclampsia and on birth weight. BJOG, 82:572. **5.** Blumenthal I (1976) Diets and diuretics in pregnancy and subsequent growth of offspring. BMJ, 2:733. **6.** Society of Actuaries (1980) 1979 Build Study. Society of Actuaries & Association of Life Assurance Medical Directors of America. **7.** Bruch H (1974) Eating Disorders. Routledge, Kegan and Paul, UK. **8.** Orbach S (1979) Fat is a feminist issue. Hamlyn, UK.

Diet and pregnancy problems
(pages 36–37)

1. Diggory PLC, Tomkinson JS (1962) Nausea and vomiting in pregnancy. L, 2:370. **2.** Speert H, Guttmacher AF (1954) Frequency and significance of bleeding in early pregnancy. JAMA, 155:712. **3.** Brandes J (1967) First trimestre nausea and vomiting as related to outcome of pregnancy. OG, 30:427. **4.** Maxwell KD, Niebyl JR (1982) Treatment of nausea and vomiting in pregnancy. *In* Drug use in pregnancy. Ed: Niebyl JR. Lea and Febiger, Philadelphia. **5.** Kloss J (1972), Back to Eden. Lifeline Books, Santa Barbara, California. **6.** King A (1955) The treatment of pregnancy nausea with a pill. OG, 6:332. **7.** Enkin M, Chalmers I (1982) Symptomatic treatment in pregnancy. *In* Effectiveness and satisfaction in ante-natal care. Clinics in Developmental Medicine 81/82, Heinemann, UK. **8.** Morrissey JF, Barreras RF (1974) Drug therapy: antacid therapy. NEJM, 290:550. **9.** Redman C (1982) Management of pre-eclampsia. *In* Effectiveness and satisfaction in ante-natal care (see 7). **10.** Wynne-Tyson J (1975) Food for a future: the ecological priority of a human diet. Davis-Poynter, London. **11.** Robinson M (1958) Salt in pregnancy. L, 1:178. **12.** Blumenthal I (1976) Diets and diuretics in pregnancy and subsequent growth of offspring. BMJ, 2:733. **13.** Rush D (1981) Nutrition services during pregnancy and birth weight: a retrospective matched pair analysis. CMAJ, 125:567. **14.** People's League of Health (1942) Nutrition of expectant and nursing mothers. CMAJ, 125:565. **15.** People's League of Health (1946) The nutrition of nursing and expectant mothers in relation to maternal and infant mortality and morbidity. JOG, 53:498.

To breast or bottle-feed?
(pages 38–39)

1. USDHEW (1979) Trends in breastfeeding among American mothers. Vital and Health Statistics Series, No.23. Department of Health, Education and Welfare, Washington. **2.** DHSS (1977) The composition of mature human breast milk. Report on Health and Social Subjects No. 12. Department of Health and Social Security, HMSO, London. **3.** Viseshakul D (1977) Breastfeeding practice of the hillside people of Thailand. JHN, 31:189. **4.** Amman AJ, Stiem ER (1966) Immunoglobulin levels in colostrum and breast milk. PSEBM, 122:1098. **5.** Menkes JH (1977) Early feeding history of children with learning disorders. DMCN, 19:169. **6.** Broad FE (1975) Further studies on the effects of infant feeding on speech quality. NZMJ, 82:373. **7.** Ironside AG, et al (1970) A survey of infantile gastro-enteritis. BMJ, 3:20. **8.** Cunningham AS (1977) Morbidity in breastfed and artificially-fed infants. JP, 90:726. **9.** Mueller M (1976) The baby killers. Oxford Committee for Famine Relief, Oxford, England. **10.** Taitz LS (1971) Over-nutrition among artificially fed infants in the Sheffield region. BMJ, 1:315. **11.** Taitz LS (1977) Weight gain and infant feeding. L, 2:712. **12.** Anderson JD (1975) Breastfeeding and cancer. SAMJ, 49:479. **13.** Rosenbloom L, Stills JA (1975) Hypernatraemic dehydration and infant mortality. ADC, 50:750. **14.** Taitz LS, Byers HD (1972) ADC, 47:257. **15.** Mettler AE (1978) The application of whey products in the babyfood industry. Unpublished paper. **16.** Reiser R, Sidelman Z (1972) Control of serum cholesterol by cholesterol in milk of the suckling rat. JN, 102:1009. **17.** Hahn P, Kirby L (1973) Immediate and late effects of premature weaning and of feeding a high-fat or high-carbohydrate diet to weaning rats. JN, 103:690. **18.** Vladian I, Reed R (1978) Adult health related to child growth and development. Harvard School of Public Health, unpublished, cited *in* P, 62:4. **19.** Davies DF, et al (1974) Food antibodies and myocardial infarction. L, 1012. **20.** War on Want (1982) Breast or bottle? International Baby Food Action Network. **21.** Chard T, Richards M (1977) Benefits and hazards of the new obstetrics. Clinics in Developmental Medicine No. 64. Heinemann, London. **22.** Jelliffe DB, Jelliffe EFP (1979) Cultural traditions and nutrition tabus related to pregnancy and lactation *in* The mother/child dyad – nutritional aspects. Ed: Hambraeus L, Sjolin S. Symposia of the Swedish Nutrition Foundation, Almqvist & Wiksell, Stockholm.

Feelings about breast feeding
(pages 40–41)

1. Kitzinger S (1979) The experience of breastfeeding. Penguin Books, London. **2.** Groddeck G (1974) The Book of the It. Vision Books. **3.** Balaskas A, Stirk J (1983) Soft Exercises. George Allen & Unwin. **4.** Iyengar BKS (1966) Light on yoga. George Allen & Unwin, London.

The birth (pages 44–45)

1. MacFarlane A (1976) The Psychology of childbirth. Fontana/Open Books, London. **2.** Kitzinger S (1981) The experience of childbirth. Pelican Books, London. **3.** Chard T, Richards M (1977) Benefits and hazards of the new obstetrics. Clinics in Developmental Medicine No. 64. Heinemann, London. **4.** Kitzinger S (1981) Some women's experience of episiotomy. National Childbirth Trust, London. **5.** Nelson MN, Enkin NW, Sigall S (1980) A randomised clinical trial of the Leboyer approach to birth. NEJM, 302:655. **6.** American Academy of Pediatrics (1981) Breastfeeding: a commentary in celebration of the International Year of the Child from the Nutrition Committee of the Canadian

References

Pediatric Society and the Committee on Nutrition of the American Academy of Pediatrics. P, 62:4. **7.** Levin B, Mackay HM, Neill A (1959) Weight gains, serum protein levels and health of breastfed and artificially fed infants. Medical Research Council, UK, Special Report No. 296. HMSO, London. **8.** Klaus HH, Kennell JH (1976) Maternal-infant bonding. C.V. Mosby. **9.** Ashford J (1977) Policies for maternity care *in* Davis J, Kitzinger S (1977) The place of birth, Oxford University Press.

Early feeding
(pages 48–49)
1. Fomon SJ, et al (1964) Milk or formula volume ingested by infants fed ad-lib. AJDC, 108:601. **2.** Hall B (1975) Changing composition of human milk and early development of an appetite control. L, 1:779. **3.** Gunther M, Stanier JE (1949) Diurnal variation in the fat content of breast milk. L, 2:235. **4.** Wright B, Fawcett J, Crow RA (1980) The development of the differences in the feeding behaviour of bottle and breastfed infants. BP, 5:1. **5.** Gunther M (1979) The nursing couple and the anti-infective qualities of fats. PNS, 38:113A. **6.** Grady E (1980) Breastfeeding a baby with a cleft of the soft palate. La Leche League International Report No. 82. **7.** Good J (1980) Breastfeeding the Down's Syndrome baby. LLI Information Sheet No. 51. **8.** Canadian Pediatric Society Committee on Nutrition (1981) Statement on feeding the low birth-weight infant. CMAJ, 124:1301. **9.** Ford J et al (1977) Influence of the heat treatment of human milk on some of its protective constituents. JP, 90:29. **10.** Liebhaber M et al (1977) Alterations of lymphocytes and of human milk after processing. JP, 91:897. **11.** La Leche League (1981) The Womanly Art of Breastfeeding. **12.** Gross SJ (1979) Vitamin E and neonatal bilirubinemia. P, 64:321.

At the breast
(pages 50–51)
1. Dyal L (1978) Breastfeeding after a caesarian birth. LLI Information Sheet No. 80. **2.** American Academy of Pediatrics (1978) Breastfeeding. A Commentary in celebration of the International Year of the Child, 1979: Statement of the Nutrition Committee of the Canadian Pediatric Society and the Committee on Nutrition of the American Academy of Pediatrics. P, 62(4).

More about breastfeeding
(pages 52–53)
1. Cahill MA, Lowman K (1982) Working and breastfeeding. LLI. **2.** La Leche League International (1972). Nursing an adoptive baby. **3.** Fomon SJ, Strauss RG (1978) Nutrient deficiencies in breastfed infants. NEJM, 299:7. **4.** Macmillian J et al (1976) Iron in breast milk. P, 58(5):686. **5.** Lakdawala DR, Widdowson EM (1977) Vitamin D in human milk. L, 1:167.

Diet and breastfeeding
(pages 54–57)
1. Winberg J, et al (1976) The case for breastfeeding. CMRO, 4 (Suppl. 1):9) **2.** Thomson AM, et al (1970) The energy cost of human lactation. BJN, 24:565. **3.** Deodhar AD, Ramakrishnan CV (1960) Studies on human lactation. JTP, Sept. 1960:44. **4.** Gyorgy P (1971) Biochemical aspects. AJCN, 24:970. **5.** Reiser R, Sidelman Z (1972) Control of serum cholesterol homeostasis by cholesterol in the milk of the suckling rat. JN, 102:1009. **6.** Gunther M, Stanier JE (1949) Diurnal variation in the fat content of breast milk. L, 2:235. **7.** Gopalan C, Belvady B (1961) Nutrition and lactation. FP, 20 (Suppl. 7) :177. **8.** Guggenheim KY (1981) Nutrition and nutritional diseases: the evolution of concepts. Collamore Press, Heath and Co., Lexington. **9.** Goel KM et al (1976) Florid and subclinical rickets among immigrant children in Glasgow. L, 1:1141. **10.** Bachrachs S, et al (1979) An outbreak of Vitamin D deficiency in a susceptible population. P, 64:871. **11.** Hurley LS (1980) Developmental Nutrition. Prentice-Hall, New Jersey. **12.** Walker ARP, et al (1978) Studies in human mineral metabolism, I. Biochem. J, 42:452. **13.** Walker AR, et al (1972) The influence of numerous pregnancies and lactations on bone dimensions in South African Bantu and Caucasian mothers. CS, 42:189. **14.** Murray MJ et al (1978) The effect of iron status of Nigerian mothers on that of their infants at birth and six months. BJN, 39:627. **15.** Saarinen UM, et al (1977) Iron absorption in infants: high bioavailability of breast milk iron as indicated by the extrinsic tag method. JP, 91(1):36. **16.** Winberg J, et al (1976) The case for breastfeeding, CMRO 4 (Suppl. 1):9. **17.** Lust J (1974) The herb book. Bantam Books, New York

Early bottle-feeding
(pages 58–61)
1. Wright P, et al (1980) The development of the differences in the feeding behaviour of bottle and breastfed infants. BP, 5:1 **2.** Bruch H (1974) Eating Disorders. Routledge, Kegan and Paul. **3.** Gerrard JW, et al (1973) Cows' milk allergy: prevalence and manifestations. APS, Suppl. 234. **4.** American Academy of Pediatrics (1979) Fluoride supplementation: revised dosage schedule. P, 63:150. **5.** La Rue A (1960) Effects of acidified milk pathogens. CMAJ, 5 November. **6.** Myles M (1958) A Textbook for Midwives. E & S Livingstone, Edinburgh. **7.** Friedman WF (1967) Vitamin D as a cause of supravalvular aortic stenosis syndrome. AHJ, 73:718.

The mother's well-being
(pages 62–63)
1. Welburn V (1980) Postnatal Depression. Fontana Books, London. **2.** Perez A, et al (1971) Timing and sequence of resuming ovulation and menstruation after childbirth. PS, 25:491. **3.** Applegate WW, et al (1979) Physiological and psychological effect of Vitamins E and B6 on women taking oral contraceptives. IJVNR, 49:43.

Your baby's digestion
(pages 64–65)
1. Jakobsson I, Lindberg T (1978) Cows' milk as a cause of infantile colic in breastfed babies. L, 2,437.

Early feeding problems
(pages 66–67)
1. Tripp JH, Wilmers, MJ, Wharton BA (1977) Gastro-enteritis: a continuing problem of child health. L, 2,233. **2.** Werner D (1979) Where there is no doctor: a village health care handbook. Macmillan Tropical Community Health Care Manuals, London. **3.** WHO (1981) Use of locally available drinking water for preparation of oral rehydration salt (ORS) solution. Diarrhoeal Disease Control Programme, WHO.

Weight gain
(pages 68–69)
1. Poskitt EME, Cole TJ (1977) Do fat babies stay fat? BMJ, 1:7. **2.** Poskitt EME, Cole TJ (1977) Nature, nurture and childhood overweight. BMJ, 1:603. **3.** Brook CGD (1972) Evidence for a sensitive period in adipose-cell replication in man. L, 2:624. **4.** Bray GA, York DA (1971) PR, 51:598.

Growth and development
(pages 72–73)
1. Winnicott D (1964) The child, the family and the outside world. Pelican Books, London. **2.** Thomson B, Rahman AK (1967) Infant feeding and child care in a West African village. JTP, 124. **3.** Sjolin S, Hofvander Y, Hillervik C (1977) APS, 66:505. **4.** Mackarness R (1976) Not all in the mind. Pan Books, London. **5.** Oski FA, Landaw SA (1980) Inhibition of iron absorption from human milk by baby food. AJDC, 134:459. **6.** Bruch H (1978) The golden cage: the enigma of anorexia nervosa. Open Books, London.

A new balance
(pages 78–79)
1. Leach P (1979) Baby and Child. Michael Joseph, London. **2.** Davis C (1939) Results of the self-selection of diets by young children. CMAJ, 4:257. **3.** Newburn E (1973) Sugar, sugar substitutes and non-caloric sweetening agents. IDJ, 23:328.

Illness and diet
(pages 80–81)
1. Weinberg ED (1966) Roles of metallic iron in host-parasite interactions. BR, 30:136. **2.** Weinberg ED (1971) Roles of iron in host-parasite interactions. JID, 124:401. **3.** Bleumink E (1970) Food allergy: the chemical nature of the substances eliciting symptoms. World Review of Nutrition and Dietetics 12:505. **4.** Feingold B (1975) Hyperkinesis and learning disabilities linked to artificial flavours and colors AJN, 75:797.

Dietary deficiencies
(pages 82–83)
1. Arthurton MN (1977) Some medical problems of Asian immigrant children. Journal of Maternal and Child Health, August:316. **2.** Meyer WW (1972) Calcifications of the carotid syphon – a common finding in infancy and childhood. ADC, 47:355. **3.** US White House Conference on Children (1970) Profiles of children. US Government Printing Office, Washington DC. **4.** Owen M (1976) Nutritional status of pre-school children. SMJ, 69:257. **5.** Hambridge KM, et al (1976) Zinc nutrition of pre-school children in the Head-Start Program. AJCN, 29:734. **6.** Sherman AR et al (1977) Inter-relationships between dietary iron and tissue zinc and copper levels and serum lipids in rats. Proceedings of the Society for Experimental Biology and Medicine, 156(3):396. **7.** Schroeder HA (1973) The trace elements and man. Devin-Adair Company, Connecticut. **8.** Food and Nutrition Board (1974) Proposed fortification policy for cereal-grain products. National Academy of Sciences, National Research Council, Washington DC. **9.** American Academy of Pediatrics (1979) Fluoride supplementation: revised dosage schedule. P, 63:150.

Supplements, rhythms and routines
(pages 84–85)
1. Davis A (1981) Let's have healthy children. New American Library. **2.** Schroeder HA (1973) The trace elements and man. Devin-Adair Company, Connecticut. **3.** Luce G (1971) Biological rhythms in psychiatry and medicine. US Dept. Health, Education and Welfare. Public Health Service Publication No. 2088. *republished as* Biological rhythms in human and animal physiology, Dover Publications, New York, 1972. **4.** Gunther M, Stanier JE (1949) Diurnal variation in the fat content of breast milk. L, 2:235. **5.** Wright B, et al (1980) The development of the differences in the feeding behaviour of bottle and breastfed infants. BP, 5:1. **6.** Helbrugge T, et al (1964) Circadian periodicity of physiological functions in different stages of infancy and childhood. Annals of the New York Academy of Science, 117:361. **7.** Brody S (1956) Patterns of mothering. International Universities Press, New York. **8.** Ainsworth MD, Bell SM (1969) Some contemporary patterns in mother-infant interactions. *In* Ambrose A (1969) Stimulation in early infancy. Academic Press, London. **9.** Winnicott D (1964) The child, the family and the outside world. Pelican Books, London.

Index

abnormalities, physical, *see* congenital defects
abortion
    spontaneous 25
    stimulation of 29
active birth 39, 44
adaptation, maternal 11, 36
addiction 9, 13, 24, 25, 78
    see also alcohol, drugs
additives, *see* food additives
adopted baby, breastfeeding of 53, 66
afterbirth, *see* placenta
alcohol
    effects of 9, 13, 24, 25, 57
    see also addiction
allergy
    to cows' milk 56, 58, 65, 66, 73, 77, 81
    to other substances 58, 65, 66, 73, 81
    see also asthma
aluminum hydroxide 36
alveoli 54
amino acids 26, 56

Index

amniotic fluid 11
anemia 31, 56
  see also iron
anesthesia, in delivery 39, 44
animal fats 19, 27
  foods, need for 14, 16
anorexia 13, 33
antacids 36
antibiotics 81
antibodies 26, 38
anxiety, *see* stress
appetite
  and breastfeeding 54, 55
  in babies 73
  in children 80
  in pregnancy 10, 13, 35
  see also anorexia, diet, hunger, illness and diet, overeating, undereating
artificial coloring and flavors, *see* food additives
ascorbic acid, *see* Vitamin C
aspirin 80–81
asthma 81
atherosclerosis 27, 78, 82

baby
  blues, *see* post-natal depression
  development of self-confidence in 72, 85
  growth and development of 68–69, 72–73, 74, 75
  nutrition notes of 88–89
  obesity in 68
  size of 34
  see also allergy, birth, diet, digestion, feeding, weight
bacteria, intestinal 54, 57
balanced diet, *see* diet, balanced
Barrie, Professor Herbert 77
beriberi 56
beta blockers 37
beverages, *see* drinks
bile 49
  see also jaundice
bilirubin 49
  see also jaundice
birth 44–45
  active 39, 44
  at home 45
  attitude to 44
  caesarian section 37, 39
  control, *see* contraception
  defects, *see* congenital defects
  in hospital 39, 44, 45, 84
  natural, *see* natural childbirth
blastocyst 10
bleeding, intestinal 77
blood
  analysis 13
  cholesterol levels in 56
  exchange of, in placenta 10, 11
  pressure 37, 84
  sugar levels 13, 22–23, 26
  variations in samples 84
  volume in pregnancy 11
  see also anemia, hypertension
body fat 68
  temperature 84
bonding 38, 45
bottle-feeding
  and physical contact 43, 58, 61
  changing to breastfeeding from 61, 66
  hygiene and 43, 59, 60–61
  preparations for 43, 58–59, 60–61
  size of nipples 59, 60
  weaning from 74, 76
  see also by-the-clock feeding, demand-feeding, digestion, formulas, weaning
bowel movements 66–67
  see also constipation, diarrhea, digestion, stools
bran 15, 27
bras, breastfeeding models 40
bread, additives in 27
  see also bran, food, refined foods
breast cancer, *see* cancer
breast milk
  bank 49
  composition 38, 48, 53, 54–55, 56, 57, 84
  drugs and 55
  drying up of 68, 73, 75
  expressing of 40, 52, 53, 55, 73
  making of 54–55
  vitamins in 55, 56
  see also colostrum
breastfeeding
  advantages of 38–39, 84
  attitudes to 38, 40
  caesarian section and 43, 50
  and conception 63
  diet and 12, 32, 52, 54–55, 62
  drugs and 48, 55
  guidance for 40, 73
  hospital routine and 39
  illness and 43, 51
  liquid intake and 57
  phasing out 53, 74, 76

position for 50
in pregnancy 73
preparations for 42, 52, 53
stress and 68, 69
supplements and 53
  see also by-the-clock feeding, demand-feeding, weaning
breasts
  care of 42, 51
  engorgement of 51
  massaging 42, 51
  mastitis 51
  shape of and feeding 41
  see also breast milk, breastfeeding
brewer's yeast, *see* yeast
bronchitis 77
Bruch, Professor Hilda 35, 73
burping 52, 59, 65
butter 14, 16, 19
  see also fats
by-the-clock-feeding 48, 50, 58, 73, 80, 84–85
  see also bottle-feeding, breastfeeding, demand-feeding

cadmium 9, 83
caesarian section 37, 39, 50, 63
  breastfeeding and 50
caffeine 9, 13, 24–25, 57
  content chart 25
  see also chocolate, cocoa, coffee, tea
calcium
  carbonate 36
  foods rich in 9, 30
  in milk 30, 57
  requirements of baby 30
  requirements of mother 30
calories 32, 54
Campbell and MacGillivray 33
candy, *see* sugar
carbohydrates 15, 26
caries, *see* dental decay, teeth
celiac disease 81
cereals 27, 68, 83
  for weaning 72–73, 74–75, 76–77
cheese 16
chemicals, *see* food additives, fertilizers
chewing 23, 76–77
childbirth, *see* birth
chocolate 21, 25, 57
  see also caffeine, sugar
cholesterol 27, 39, 56
cigarettes, *see* smoking
cleft palate, effect on feeding 48
clock, feeding by the
  see by-the-clock feeding
Cochrane, Dr W. 29
cocoa, *see* chocolate
cod-liver oil 57, 82
coffee 9, 24–25, 57
  see also caffeine
colic 65
  see also crying
colon, *see* bowel, digestion
colostrum 37, 38, 48, 49, 54, 56
conception
  diet before 7–9, 35
  effect of malnutrition on 7–9
congenital defects 8–9, 33
  see also spina bifida
constipation 27, 54, 66, 80–81
contact, mother-baby, *see* bonding
contraception 9, 28, 63
  resuming after the birth 63
contraceptive pill,
  and vitamin needs 63
cookbooks 23, 96
cooking oils 19
  see also fats, fatty spreads
copper 9
cows' milk
  iron content of 82
  unsuitability for new baby 58
  see also allergy
cramps 59
cravings 19
crying, reasons for 65, 68
curds 64–65

dairy products, *see* butter, cheese, milk
Davis, Adelle 84
Davis, Dr Clara 78, 80
deficiency diseases,
  see malnutrition
dehydration 67, 81
  prevention of 67
  see also rehydration salts
demand-feeding 50, 58, 84–85
  see also by-the-clock feeding
dental decay 15, 78, 83
depression, *see* post-natal depression
Determination of Sex, (Dr Leopold Schenk) 9
diabetes 12, 15, 21, 34, 78
diarrhea in babies and children 54, 60, 66–67, 77, 80–81
  suitable foods during 80–81
  treatment of 67, 81
  see also rehydration salts

diet
  balanced 8–9, 12–23, 54–55, 62, 77, 78–79, 80
  and breastfeeding 12, 54–55
  changing the 15, 34–35
  in lactation 54
  in pregnancy 8–9, 12–23
  prior to conception 8–9
  unbalanced, effect of 15
  see also anorexia, macrobiotic diet, obesity, overweight, underweight, vegetarianism, weight gain
dietary laws, religious 24
dietary fiber, *see* fiber
dieting 13, 15, 37
digestion
  baby's 64–65
  in pregnancy 10
disease, resistance to 8
diuretics 33, 37
diverticulitis 27
Down's syndrome 48
drinks
  for babies 68, 77
  for children 79
  in pregnancy 25
  see also alcohol, cocoa, coffee, milk, sugar, tea
drugs
  avoidance of 9, 55
  effect on feeding 48
  see also addiction

E. Coli 54
eating disorders 13, 15, 58, 73
  habits 13
  see also anorexia, overeating, undereating
Ebbs, Tisdall and Scott 12
eclampsia 37
eczema 81
  see also allergy
edema 3, 37
egg, human, *see* ovum
eggs 14, 16, 57
  see also animal foods
embryo, growth and development of 10–11
  see also fetus
emergency formula, *see* formulas, home-made emergency
emotional eating disorders, *see* eating disorders
endosperm of grain 15
enema 44, 45
engorgement, *see* breasts, engorgement of
Enkin, Professor Murray 36
enteritis, *see* gastroenteritis
enzymes 8, 30, 64
episiotomy 39, 45, 62, 63
essential fatty acids, *see* fatty acids
excrement, *see* stools
exercise 9, 34, 62, 63
expressing, *see* milk

Fallopian tubes 8, 10
fast foods 23, 78
fasting in children 80
fat, *see* body fat
fathers
  attitudes to breastfeeding 41
  diet of, prior to conception 9
  presence at birth 41, 45
fats
  consumption of 15, 27
  for cooking 19
  in milk 13, 56
  saturated and unsaturated 19
fatty acids 19, 27
  spreads 27
  see also cooking oils
Fawcett and Wright 58
feasting, *see* overeating
feeding, *see* breastfeeding, bottle-feeding, by-the-clock, demand-feeding, weaning
Feingold, Dr Ben 81
fertilizers, use of 22
fetus, growth and development of 10–11
fevers 80
fiber 15, 26–27, 80
fish 16, 22, 57
  see also recipes
flavors, *see* artificial coloring and flavors
fluid retention, *see* edema
fluoride 83
fluorosis 83
folic acid 28–29, 37, 63
Fomon, Professor Samuel 53
food
  additives 22, 81
  frozen 18
  highly processed 13, 14, 15, 20, 22, 37
  raw 14, 18
  unrefined 54, 78, 84
  see also allergy, bottle-feeding, breastfeeding, diet, feeding, weaning

forceps delivery 25
formula-feeding, *see* bottle-feeding, formulas
formulas
  changing 61, 65, 66
  composition of 38–39
  home-made emergency 60–61
  non-milk 58
  overconcentrated 61, 68
  overdilution 69
  preparation of 58–59, 60–61, 68
  use of in Third World 38
  see also allergies, bottle-feeding, by-the-clock feeding, demand-feeding
frozen foods, *see* food
fruits, *see* vegetables and fruits

galactose 66
galactosemia 66
Gartner, Lawrence 49
gastric juices 64
  see also digestion
gastroenteritis 66–67
germ, of whole grain 15
glucose 22, 26
gluten, *see* celiac disease
goitre 83
grains 14–15, 16–17, 26, 27
granola 14, 20, 76
group therapy 62
growth chart 69, 89
guidelines for a balanced diet 13–23

hair analysis 13
halva 19
handicaps, *see* congenital defects
hatha yoga, *see* yoga
headaches, *see* migraine
heart conditions, diet as factor in 15, 21
heartburn 36
Hemminki and Starfield 28
hemoglobin 30–31
hemorrhoids 27
herbal remedies 36
  see also tea, herbal
high blood pressure, *see* hypertension
home base, baby's recognition of 72
home, birth at 45
hormones 8, 13
hospital routines 39, 44, 84
hunger and appetite
  in pregnancy 10, 13, 33, 35
  of baby 13, 58, 84
  see also by-the-clock feeding, demand-feeding
hyperactivity 81
hypertension 33, 37

ice cream 78
  see also snacks, sugar
illness and diet 56, 66–67, 80–81
immunity proteins, *see* immunoglobulins
immunoglobulins 38, 54, 56
indigestion 36
induction of labor, *see* labor
infection, *see* diarrhea, illness and diet
insulin, *see* diabetes
intestines, *see* bowel, digestion
iodine 57, 83
iron
  and constipation 66
  deficiency 82
  foods rich in 73, 77, 82
  in milk 53, 77, 82
  in newborn's blood 45
  intake and milk consumption 57
  requirements 30–31
  supplements 31, 84

jaundice 49
jogging, *see* exercise

keep-fit, *see* exercise
kidneys
  adaptation of (to pregnancy) 11
  damage to 36
  function of 64
Kitzinger, Sheila 44
Kloss, Jethro 36

La Leche League 39, 63, 73
labor
  anesthesia in 39, 44
  hospital management of 39, 44, 84
  induction of 25, 37, 39, 44
  pain in 44
  see also birth
lactation, *see* breastfeeding, breast milk
lactobacillus bifidus 54
lactoferrin 53, 57
lactose 54
  intolerance 30, 66
  see also galactosemia
laxatives, use of 80
  see also constipation
lead poisoning 9, 84
Leboyer, Frederick 44
Lechtat 24
legumes 14, 16–17, 27

95

let-down reflex, see reflexes
Let's Have Healthy Children (Adelle Davis) 84
Leibig, J. von 39
Lind, T. 31
liquid intake, during breastfeeding 57
  see also breastfeeding
liver
  carbohydrate store in 26
  in diet 84
love-making 8, 62
low-birth-weight babies 8, 27, 49, 69

MacGillivray and Campbell 33
McCarrison, Robert 15
macrobiotic diet 15, 19
magnesium 54, 57
  salts 36
malnutrition 82–83
  effect on conception 8
  symptoms of 82–83
margarine 14, 19
  enriched 57, 82
massage 42
  of baby's abdomen 66
mastitis 51
maternal adaptation, see adaptation, maternal
meals, see diet, feeding, weaning
meat 14, 16–17
  see also animal foods
meconium 49, 64
medication, see drugs
meditation, see yoga
mealtimes 78
Mellanby, Professor Edward 12
metabolism 26, 32, 36, 56, 64–65
methyldopa 37
Metropolitan Life Insurance Company
  table of desirable weights 34
micro-nutrients, see minerals, vitamins
midwife 45
migraine 37
milk
  amount drunk by babies 77, 82
  high intake of 12, 77, 82
  humanized 39
  minerals in 39, 57, 82
  and tooth decay 61
  unmodified 77
  vitamin enriched 39, 57, 82
  see also allergy, cows' milk, breast milk, formulas, lactose
mineral deficiencies 82
  supplements 30–31, 57, 39, 84
minerals in common foods 30–31
  in milk 30
miso 17, 19
mongolism, see Down's syndrome
Montgomery's tubercles 54
Montreal Diet Dispensary 12, 27
morning sickness 36–37
mother
  and baby, separation of 44, 45
  bonding of baby to 38
  nutrition notes of 86–87
  well-being of 62–63
  working 40, 53
  see also adaptation (maternal), breastfeeding
Mott, Francis 10
Myles, Maggie 60

naso-gastric tube, feeding by 49
natural childbirth 39, 44
nausea 36–37
  see also morning sickness
nicotine, see smoking
night-blindness 82
night-feedings 48, 63, 69
nipples
  for bottle-feeding 59, 61, 69
  of breasts 42
  inverted 42
  lubrication of 42
  massage of 42
  sore 51
  teasing with 50
non-nutritive sucking, see sucking (non-nutritive)
nursing supplementer 53, 61
nutrients
  see carbohydrates, fats, protein, minerals, vitamins
nuts 9, 14, 16–17, 27

obesity 33, 34, 68, 73
  see also weight, overeating
Odent, Michel 44
oils for cooking 14, 19
  see also fats
oral contraception, see contraceptive pill
oral salts 67, 81
Osofsky, Dr. H. J: 26
overeating, compulsive 13, 15, 32–33, 62, 80
overfeeding, of infants 68
overweight 12, 33, 34–35
ovulation 63

ovum 8
oxytocin 8

pancreas 23
pesticides, use of 22
phosphorus, 30
phototherapy 49
pica, see cravings
piles, see hemorrhoids
polio 54
placenta
  beliefs about 10
  function of 10–11
plaque (of teeth) 79
post-natal
  depression (PND) 62
  exercises 62–63
posture 41
potassium 57
pre-eclampsia,
  see toxemia
pregnancy 7–45
  see also alcohol, conception, cravings, diet, drugs, exercise, morning sickness, nutrients, smoking, taboos, weight gain in
premature babies 27, 48, 49
pre-natal exercise, see exercise
Price, Weston 15
processed foods
  see foods
protein
  deficiency 26–27
  in milk 56
  need for 26–27, 37
  sources of 26–27
  supplements 26–27, 56
psychotherapy 62

Rahman, A.K. 72
rashes, see allergy
raw food, see food
RDAs (recommended daily allowances) 12
recipes
  baked apples 18
  baked trout 16
  brown rice 15
  everday salad 18
  French dressing 18
  fruit and yoghurt purée 75
  nut croquettes 16
  rice and vegetable purée 75
  stir-fried vegetables 18
  sugarless muffins 79
  weaning granola 76
  white fish (steamed) 76
  wholewheat pastry 15
reflexes
  let-down 48
  rooting 48
  sucking 48
regression, to breast or bottle 78
rehydration salts 67, 81
relaxation 42, 63
  see also exercise, stress
religion, see dietary laws
rest, see relaxation
rhythms 58, 84–85
rice, see recipes
rickets 56, 57, 82
rooting reflex, see reflexes
routines 78, 84–85
  see also mealtimes
Rush, Professor David 26, 37
rusks 74

safflower seed oil 27
salads, see vegetables and fruit, recipes
salt 14, 20, 37, 78
  iodized 83
saturated fats, see fats
Schenk, Dr Leopold 9
Schroeder, Dr Henry 83
Scott, Tisdall and Ebbs 12
scurvy 29, 82
seeds 9, 14, 16–17, 27
sesame butter 14, 17
sex of baby
  effect of diet on 9
Shenolikar, Dr. I. 30
shields, for inverted nipples 42
shigella 54
sleeping, position of baby for 65
smoking, effects of 9, 15, 24–25, 55
  see also addiction
snacks 78
sodium 9
  bicarbonate 36
  citrate 60
solids, introduction of, see weaning
Soranus 9
soybean 14, 16, 17
  paste, see miso
sperm production, effect of diet on 8
spina bifida 28
starch 26
Starfield and Hemminki 28
sterility 9

sterilizing, see bottle-feeding
Stolkowski, Professor 9
stools
  excretion of 66–67
  watery 66–67
  see also constipation, diarrhea, meconium
storage of feedings 59
stress 8–9, 22, 35, 37, 62–63, 65, 66, 68, 82
stretching 9, 41, 63
  see also exercise, relaxation
stroke 27
sucking 48, 52
  impairment of 44, 52
  non-nutritive 48, 49
sugar 14–15, 20–21, 61, 66, 74, 77, 78–79
  see also glucose
sugar water 48, 49
sunflower oil 19, 27
  seeds 19
sunlight, and Vitamin D 57, 82
supplementer, nursing 53, 61
supplements
  in baby's diet 61, 77, 84
  in bottle-feeding 61
  in breastfeeding 53
  in pregnancy 9, 28–29, 37
  natural 84
  overdosing 61

taboos 24–25, 63, 73
tantrums, see temper tantrums
Taylor, D. J. 31
tea 24–25, 57
  herbal 25, 36, 57
teeth
  cleaning of 77
  decay of 61, 78, 83
  development of 77, 79
  loss of 30, 78–79
teething biscuits 74
temper tantrums 85
tension
  relieving 62–63
  see also colic, stress
Textbook for Midwives (Maggie Myles) 60
thiamin, see vitamins, specific (B's)
Third World, diet in 26, 57
  gastroenteritis in 67
  weaning in 72
  see also malnutrition
Thomson, A. M. 31
thyroid 83
tiredness 62–63
Tisdall, Ebbs and Scott 12
tobacco, see smoking
toilet training 85
toothbrush, see teeth
toxemia 25, 33, 34, 37

umbilical
  cord, clamping of 39, 44, 45
undereating 13
  see also anorexia, weight
underfeeding 68–69
underweight 34–35
  see also weight
unrefined foods, see food
unsaturated fats, see fats
urine 64
uterus 10, 44

vegans 56
vegetables and fruit 57, 82, 84
  see also recipes, roughage, vitamins
vegetarians 16, 28, 57
vitamin
  deficiencies 56–57, 82
  food sources of 28–29, 36, 56–57, 77, 82
  function of 28, 80
  natural/synthetic 84
  requirements 26, 36, 56–57
  supplements 9, 28–29, 37, 39, 49, 53, 56, 82, 84
vitamins, specific
  A 13, 28, 56, 61, 77, 82, 84
  Bs 9, 28, 36, 56, 63, 84
  C 9, 12, 13, 18, 24, 29, 56, 61, 63, 77, 80, 82, 84
  D 28, 53, 56, 57, 61, 77, 82, 84
  E 9, 49, 84
  folic acid 28–29, 37, 63
vomiting
  in babies 65, 77, 80
  in pregnancy, see morning sickness
  see also diarrhea, illness and diet, nausea

Walker, Professor A. R. 30
water
  for baby 59, 64, 65, 66, 68
  contaminated 67
  fluoridation of 59, 83
  retention, see edema
  spring and bottled 37, 57, 59
weaning
  from bottle 76–77
  from breast 76–77

foods, manufactured 74
granola 76
in Third World 72
program, flexible 74–75, 76–77, 85
recommended age for 72–73, 74, 85
premature 71, 72–73
weighing of baby 69
weight
  adjustment after birth 62
  and bottle-fed baby 68
  and breastfed baby 68
  gain in pregnancy 32–33
  gain, of baby 68–69, 85
  loss 32, 66
  low-birth-weight 69
  of newborn baby 37, 69
  overweight baby 33, 68–69
  table of desirable weights 34
  and toxemia 37
  underweight baby 68–69
well-being, of mother 62–63
wheat, digestion of 81
  see also celiac disease, gluten
wheat germ 15, 57, 84
whey 64
whole grains 9, 14–15, 83
wholewheat pastry 15
Widdowson, Professor Elsie 57
winding, see burping
Winnicott, Dr Donald 85
womb, see uterus
working mother, see mother
World Health Organization 31
Wright and Fawcett 58

yang foods 9, 24
yeast, brewer's 84
Yerushalmy, Professor 25
yin foods 9, 24
yin/yang system 9, 24
yoga 9, 41, 62
Yudkin, Professor John 20

Zen macrobiotics 19, 23, 24
  see also macrobiotic diet
zinc 9, 57, 82, 83, 84
  deficiency 82–83

Useful Addresses

American Academy of Husband-Coached Childbirth
P.O. Box 5224, Department CB
Sherman Oaks, CA 91413

American College of Home Obstetrics
664 N. Michigan Avenue, Suite 600
Chicago, IL 60611

American Society for Psychoprophylaxis in Obstetrics Inc.
1411 K Street, Suite 200
Washington DC 20005

Association for Childbirth at Home International
1675 Monte Cristo Street
Cerritos, CA 90701

Caesarians/Support, Education and Concern Inc.
22 Forest Road
Framingham, MA 01701

Home-Oriented Maternity Experience (HOME)
511 New York Avenue
Takoma Park, Washington DC. 20012

La Leche League International
9616 Mineapolis Avenue
Franklin Park, IL 60131

Maternity Center
48 E. 92nd Street
New York, NY 10028

Resources in Human Nurturing International
3885 Forrest Street
P.O. Box 6861
Denver, CO 80206